CORONAVIRUS
& ITS IMPACT ON
THE WORLD ECONOMY

A. V. Narayanmurthy

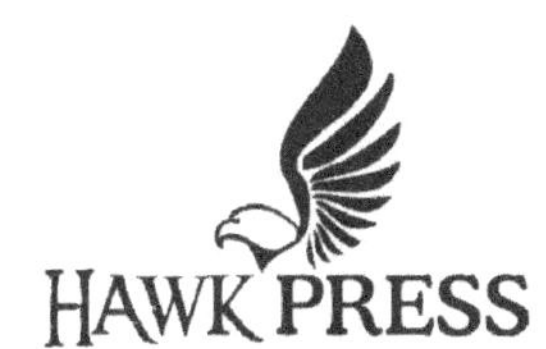

HAWK PRESS

Published by

Hawk Press
4836/24, Ansari Road, Daryaganj
New Delhi – 110 002
Phones : 9643330713, 91-11-23278618, 91-11-35676207
E-mail: thehawkpress@gmail.com
www.thehawkpress.com

Contents

Preface

China's economic growth expected to slow to 4.5% in the first quarter of 2020 – the slowest pace since the financial crisis, according to a Reuters poll of economists. As China grapples with the coronavirus, the economic damage is mounting around the world.

Second, in the current wave, the marking of containment zone has been less strict. In cities, the government has asked civil authorities to adopt micro-containment: with perhaps just a floor or a house defined as a containment zone. If there is no effective monitoring in micro-containment zones, containing the virus becomes a challenge. Earlier, an entire apartment or area would be made a containment zone, reducing the chances of transmission of the virus. Now, central teams have red-flagged the fact that high-risk contacts in workplace, social and family settings were not investigated and listed in Maharashtra, resulting in a surge. This is happening across the country.

Coronaviruses (CoV) are a large family of viruses that cause illness ranging from the common cold to more severe diseases such as Middle East Respiratory Syndrome (MERS-CoV) and Severe Acute Respiratory Syndrome (SARS-CoV). A novel coronavirus (nCoV) is a new strain that has not been previously identified in humans.

China has become an indispensable part of global business since the 2003 SARS outbreak. It's grown into the world's factory, churning out products such as the iPhone and driving demand for commodities like oil and copper. The country also boasts hundreds of millions of wealthy consumers who spend big on luxury products, tourism and cars. China's economy accounted for roughly 4% of world GDP in 2003; it now makes up 16% of global output.

Globalization has encouraged companies to build supply chains that cut across national borders, making economies much more interconnected. The major central banks have used up much of the ammunition they would typically deploy to fight economic downturns since the 2008 financial crisis, and global debt levels have never been higher. Rising nationalism may make it harder to coordinate a worldwide response, if that's required.

The global economy could suffer the longer China stays in low gear. It has been hampered by both the outbreak and its own containment efforts, a process that has cut off workers from their jobs and factories from their raw materials. The result is a slowdown that is already slashing traffic along the world's shipping lines and leading to forecasts of a sharp fall in production of everything from cars to smartphones.

Considering China's impact on the world economy, China will not be off limits to future investment forever. Instead, there will be wariness and unbridled caution for the foreseeable future. Businesses will seek alternatives to avoid commercial and liability issues.

In the best case, returning to normal is not a reasonable expectation in the short term. In the long term, China must take all steps necessary to demonstrate its commitment to transparency regarding all factors relating to the virus. In today's economy, there are many alternatives for trade and investment and China must recognize that its global trade partners need regular and repeated reassurances. Additionally, China will need to inject substantial financial incentives into the economy to balance against commercial and optical risks.

The number of COVID-19 cases, and the resulting death toll, will only continue to rise in countries unable to properly prevent the virus' spread, care for and support the sick, and conduct comprehensive vaccination campaigns. PIH continues to advocate for equitable global COVID-19 vaccination distribution, especially considering only 0.9% of people in low-income countries have received at least one dose of a COVID-19 vaccine compared to 45% of people in high-income countries.

This book gives us a panoramic and synthetic overview of our current crisis. By focusing on finance and business, this book sets the pandemic story in a frame that casts a sobering new light on how unprepared the world was to fight the crisis, and how deep the ruptures in our way of living and doing business are.

— *Editor*

1

Introduction

In 2020, COVID-19 spread to almost all countries and affected more than 50 million people around the world. The COVID-19 crisis has governments around the world operating in a context of radical uncertainty, and faced with difficult trade-offs given the health, economic and social challenges it raises. Within the first three months of 2020, the novel coronavirus developed into a global pandemic. Schools and universities were closed in spring 2020 for more than one billion students of all ages. More than half of the world's population has experienced a lockdown with strong containment measures – the first time in history that such measures are applied on such a large scale.

Beyond the health and human tragedy of COVID-19, it is now widely recognised that the pandemic triggered the most serious economic crisis since World War II. All economic sectors are affected by disrupted global supply chains, weaker demand for imported goods and services, a drop in international tourism, a decline in business travel, and most often a combination of these.

Chinese manufacturing cities such as Wuhan, the epicenter of the outbreak, are intimately entangled with the supply chains of the entire world. That means that both the disease and the containment measures enacted to control it (take, for example, the quarantine still in place for 70 million people) will have a dramatic effect on businesses across disparate industries.

Any company—including Apple and Walmart—that brings things in from China has to worry about production and distribution slowdowns. That's partly because supply chains are less linear than they sound. Production networks often have complex interrelationships that go back and forth across borders. An American retailer might contract with only one Chinese company, but that entity in turn might act like a general contractor, pulling in components from many sources or farming out work to a changing list of factories. In 2018, for instance, more than 1,000 facilities were involved in some way with the making of Apple products.

Meanwhile, exporters—such as Brazilian ranchers and Chilean winemakers—are facing a massive drop in Chinese demand. Inside China, the economic decline is expanding beyond the manufacturing sectors; even a media company said it was laying off 500 workers because of the epidemic.

What makes this all so strange is that a mosaic of facts is known about the economic consequences of coronavirus, but the arrival of those consequences outside China will be delayed, and their magnitude is uncertain. It doesn't help that experts inside and outside China have questioned the reliability of the country's official statistics for years. And local reporting provides reasons to doubt coronavirus numbers as well.

What Target executives are worried about today will actually show up for shoppers in April. You might think that financial markets, at least, would be "pricing in" the problems, but share prices are at record highs. Coronavirus has likely already dealt many of its economic blows—and now those disruptions will trickle through the networks that connect China to the rest of the global economy.

Some of the effects will be material: There might be fewer items on store shelves, some prices might rise, product development could slow down. But some of the impact, and an additional source of lag, will come from the data describing the reality of the past two months, much of which has yet to be tabulated. Companies and governments need statistics to understand what's happening in the world. The U.S. government, for example, maintains a complex data-gathering operation: the Bureau of Economic Analysis, the Bureau of Labor Statistics, certain survey programs of the Census, the National Agricultural Statistics Service, the Economic Research Service, and many others. The data that these organizations publish take time to reflect on-the-ground commerce. Under normal conditions, this may not be significant. But when the economy suffers a globe-altering shock, statistical windows on the world can be dangerously out of step with reality.

For now, the data points that can be marshaled to make sense of the macroeconomic picture are not good. Chinese oil demand was down 20 percent earlier this month, "probably the largest demand shock the oil market has suffered since the global financial crisis of 2008 to 2009, and the most sudden since the Sept. 11 attacks," as *Bloomberg* put it. With some huge Chinese cities under varying versions of lockdown, the total number of cars and trucks on the road has fallen. Factories are not running at full capacity either. Pollution near Shanghai, a reliable and hard-to-fake indicator of economic activity, has plummeted, according to Morgan Stanley. Container ships are sailing with smaller than normal cargo loads. Prices for bulk carriers that move iron ore and coal have collapsed. One analyst told the *Financial*

Times that the coronavirus "will have a bigger impact on the global tech supply chain than SARS and creates more uncertainty than the U.S.-China trade war."

That very trade war led some companies to move their supply chains to other Asian countries, but China remains the beating heart of manufacturing and assembly for the world's goods. "Suddenly, all supply chains seem vulnerable because so many Chinese supply chains within supply chains within supply chains rely on each other for parts and raw materials," Rosemary Coates, a supply-chain consultant, wrote in the trade journal *Logistics Management.* "That tiny valve that is inside a motor that you are sourcing for your U.S.-made product is made in China. So are the rare earth elements you require to manufacture magnets and electronics." The impacts may also vary widely from province to province and even factory to factory based on how local governments regulate their regions, CNBC's Beijing bureau chief, Eunice Yoon, noted.

The slow industrial march out of China has also left some industries, like toy making, with depleted inventories. Companies that spent last year building new production networks in other Asian countries are more resilient in the long term, but at this particular moment, they may not have enough product to sell. Less predictable secondary effects have cropped up too. As Indonesia's president called for stimulus spending to guard against an economic slowdown, the price of Indonesian garlic went up 70 percent, apparently because Chinese consumers were buying up the folk cure in bulk. Even small ripples must have some effect: In Australia, where students from China could not return to class after the summer holiday, universities pushed back their start dates, which hurt the businesses around them. The question is whether all those small problems and complications will add up to anything more serious than annoyance.

Then, consider the political ramifications of the economic slowdown. What if the coronavirus crisis slows China's economic growth enough to destabilize the Communist Party's control? Bill Bishop, a longtime China analyst, wrote that the outbreak is the closest thing "to an existential crisis for Xi [Jinping] and the Party that I think we have seen since 1989."

The coronavirus is a remarkable probe for the complex relationships that hold up today's economy. In our world, information flows much more quickly than goods. That means we can glimpse a major world event, in tweets and videos from the quarantine zone, weeks before its impact will be quantified. It is an uneasy and strange position, like knowing an earthquake has struck but not knowing whether a tsunami is on the way. One upshot for Americans is likely, though: Even if the worst of the outbreak is over—and it might not be—bad economic news may well be in our future.

2019-20 CORONAVIRUS OUTBREAK

An ongoing outbreak of coronavirus disease 2019 (COVID-19), caused by SARS-CoV-2, started in December 2019. It was first identified in Wuhan, the capital of Hubei, China.

Infection by the coronavirus is primarily through human-to-human transmission via respiratory droplets that people cough, sneeze or exhale. The incubation period is typically between 2 to 14 days. Symptoms may include fever, cough, and shortness of breath. Complications may include pneumonia and acute respiratory distress syndrome and death. There are no vaccines or specific antiviral treatments, with efforts typically aiming at managing symptoms and supportive therapy. Hand washing is recommended to prevent the disease. Anyone who is suspected of carrying the virus is advised to monitor their health for two weeks, wear a surgical mask, and seek medical advice by calling a doctor before visiting a clinic.

As of 24 February 2020, around 79,364 cases have been confirmed, including in all provinces of China and more than two dozen other countries. Of these, 11,569 cases are serious. There have been 2,619 deaths attributable to the disease, including 27 outside mainland China, surpassing that of the 2003 SARS outbreak. 24,974 people have since recovered.

A large response, both in China and globally, followed an increase in cases in mid-January 2020, bringing travel restrictions, quarantines, and curfews. Examples include the quarantine of the British cruise ship *Diamond Princess* in Japan, the curfew of over 170 million in central China, a voluntary curfew in Daegu, South Korea, and the curfew of a dozen towns with over 50,000 people in the Lombardy and Veneto regions of Italy.

The outbreak has been declared a Public Health Emergency of International Concern (PHEIC) by the World Health Organization (WHO). Airports and train stations have implemented body temperature checks, health declarations, and information signage in an attempt to identify carriers of the virus. A number of countries have issued warnings against travel to Wuhan, Hubei, or China generally.

Among the wider consequences of the outbreak are concerns about potential economic instability and the firing of several local leaders of the Chinese Communist Party for their poor response to the outbreak. Outbreak-related incidents of xenophobia and racism against people of Chinese and East Asian descent have been reported in several countries. The spread of misinformation and disinformation about the virus, primarily online, has been described as an "infodemic" by the WHO.

Overview

In late December, a cluster of pneumonia cases of unknown aetiology was reported by health authorities in Wuhan, Hubei Province, People's Republic of

China. The initial cases mostly had epidemiological links to the Huanan Seafood Wholesale Market and consequently the virus is thought to have a zoonotic origin. The China CDC reported in early January that the causative agent was a novel coronavirus (now called SARS-CoV-2), which is closely related to bat coronaviruses, pangolin coronaviruses and SARS-CoV-1. Evidence shows that the transmissibility of the coronavirus is sufficient for sustained community transmission and locally acquired cases have been reported across the world, along with several deaths.

Epidemiology

2019–20 coronavirus outbreak by country and territory

Country or territory[a]	Confirmed	Deaths	Recoveries[b]
Mainland China[c]	77,150	2,592	24,734
South Korea	763	7	18
International conveyance[d]	691	3	1
Italy	155	3	2
Japan	146	1	22
Singapore	89	0	51
Hong Kong	74	2	12
Iran	43	8	1
United States	35	0	7
Thailand	35	0	21
Taiwan	28	1	2
Australia	22	0	11
Malaysia	22	0	18
Germany	16	0	14
Vietnam	16	0	15
United Arab Emirates	13	0	3
United Kingdom	13	0	8
France	12	1	10
Macau	10	0	6
Canada	10	0	3
Philippines	3	1	2
India	3	0	3
Israel	2	0	–
Russia	2	0	2
Spain	2	0	2
Iraq	1	0	–
Lebanon	1	0	–

Sweden	1	0	–
Belgium	1	0	1
Cambodia	1	0	1
Egypt	1	0	1
Finland	1	0	1
Nepal	1	0	1
Sri Lanka	1	0	1
33 territories	79,364	2,619	24,974

Notes

1. Region where case was diagnosed. Nationality and location of original infection may vary.

2. "–" denotes that no data is currently available for that territory, not that the value is zero.

3. Includes clinically diagnosed cases and deaths from 12 February 2020 and onwards in the province of Hubei, based on medical imaging features of the pneumonia. This also includes asymptomatic cases that have been tested positive for the virus.

4. The cruise ship *Diamond Princess* is currently quarantined in Japanese territorial waters and managed by the Japanese government. However, these cases are not included in the Japanese government's official count of total confirmed cases in the country. Similarly, the World Health Organization classifies the cases as being located "on an international conveyance" instead of in Japan.

Epidemiological analysis of the outbreak has shown a probable pattern of a "mixed outbreak" – there was likely a continuous common source outbreak at the seafood market in December 2019, potentially from several zoonotic events. Following this, the epidemiologists found that the outbreak likely became a propagated source (transmitted from person to person), potentially due to the virus' ability to mutate. The earliest reported symptoms occurred on 1 December 2019 in a person who had not had any exposure to the Huanan Seafood Wholesale Market or to the remaining 40 of the first cluster detected with the new virus.

Of this first cluster, two-thirds were found to have a link with the market, which also sold live animals. Of cases that began before 1 January 2020, 55% were linked to the market. By 22 January this figure was reported to have dropped to 8.6%. Hence, as the number of cases has increased, the significance of the market has lessened.

During the early stages, the number of cases doubled approximately every seven and a half days. In early and mid-January 2020, the virus spread to other Chinese provinces, helped by the Chinese new year migration. On 20 January, China reported nearly 140 new patients, including two people in Beijing and one in Shenzhen.

The virus was soon carried to other countries by international travellers: Thailand (13 January); Japan (15 January); Macau (19 January); South Korea (20 January); Taiwan and the United States (21 January); Hong Kong (22 January);

Singapore (23 January); France, Nepal, and Vietnam (24 January); Australia and Malaysia (25 January); Canada (26 January); Cambodia (27 January); Germany (28 January); Finland, Sri Lanka, and the United Arab Emirates (29 January); India, Italy, and the Philippines (30 January); the United Kingdom, Russia, Sweden, and Spain (31 January); Belgium (4 February); Egypt (14 February); Iran (19 February); Israel and Lebanon (21 February); Iraq (22 February).

By 25 January, the number of laboratory-confirmed cases had stood at 2,062, including 2,016 in Mainland China, 7 in Thailand, 6 in Hong Kong, 5 in Macau, 5 in Australia, 4 in Malaysia, 4 in Singapore, 3 in France, 3 in Japan, 3 in South Korea, 3 in Taiwan, 3 in the United States, 2 in Vietnam, 1 in Nepal, and 1 in Sweden.

Citing 7,711 cases essentially in China and 83 cases abroad across 18 countries as of 29 January, WHO declared the outbreak to be a Public Health Emergency of International Concern on 30 January. As of 24 February, 79,364 cases have been confirmed worldwide, over 98.4% in mainland China.

On 6 February, the Chinese National Health Commission (NHC) started to change how cases were reported – asymptomatic carriers, who tested positive for the virus but did not show clinical symptoms, would no longer be included in the number of confirmed cases. This had the effect of reducing the total number of cases reported, but also meant that potentially contagious individuals were ignored in reports.

On 12 February, the Hubei government adopted a broader definition of confirmed cases, which now includes clinically diagnosed patients diagnosed by their symptoms and CT scans but without nucleic acid test, which can take days to process and delay treatment. "Using CT scans that reveal lung infection would help patients receive treatment as soon as possible and improve their chances of recovery," the provincial health commission said. This new methodology accounts for the sharp increase in Hubei's daily confirmed cases: 13,332 of the 14,840 newly confirmed cases in the province on 12 February were diagnosed clinically under the new definition.

On 20 February, the Chinese National Health Commission (NHC) changed how cases are counted again by counting only cases showing positive results through laboratory tests. The change is done as the backlog of patients who needed to be treated has since cleared. Other sources interpreted the new NHC guidelines as cancelling the previous change in how Hubei (alone) was counting confirmed cases without laboratory tests, and said NHC now distinguished counting of confirmed cases from suspected cases, requiring RT-PCR or gene sequencing for confirmation of infection, whereas suspicion of infection is based on two levels of epidemiological history and clinical symptoms.

Deaths

As of 24 February, 2,619 deaths have been attributed to COVID-19. According to China's NHC, most of those who died were older patients – about 80% of deaths recorded were from those over the age of 60, and 75% had pre-existing health conditions including cardiovascular diseases and diabetes. The case fatality rate has been estimated at around 2–3%.

The first confirmed death was a 61-year-old man on 9 January 2020 who was first admitted to a Wuhan hospital on 27 December 2019. The first death outside China occurred in the Philippines, when a 44-year-old Chinese male citizen developed severe pneumonia and died on 1 February. His companion, a 38-year-old Chinese female citizen was also confirmed to have contracted the virus, but eventually recovered. She stayed in the same hospital in Manila as her companion until her discharge on 8 February. On 8 February 2020, it was announced that a Japanese and an American died from the virus in Wuhan. They were the first non-Chinese killed by the virus. The first death outside Asia was confirmed in Paris, France, on 15 February 2020, when an 80-year-old Chinese tourist from Hubei died after being in hospital since 25 January. On 19 February 2020, two elderly Japanese citizens who had been on the *Diamond Princess* died after being hospitalised for a week after they had tested positive for the virus, while a third elderly Japanese citizen died on 23 February 2020.

A 78-year-old Italian man in Veneto died on 21 February 2020, while on the following day a 75-year-old woman died in Lombardy. As of 22 February 2020 Iran has confirmed the virus has killed six people. An Italian woman died on 23 February 2020 in Lombardy.

Estimates

On 17 January, a research group from the Imperial College London in the United Kingdom published a report giving an estimate of 1,723 cases (95% confidence interval, 427–4,471) with onset of symptoms by 12 January. This was based on the pattern of the initial spread to Thailand and Japan. They also concluded that "self-sustaining human-to-human transmission should not be ruled out", which has since been confirmed. As further cases came to light, they later recalculated that there may be 4,000 symptomatic cases in Wuhan City by 18 January (uncertainty range of 1,000 to 9,700). A Hong Kong University group has reached a similar conclusion as the earlier study, with additional detail on transport within China.

Based on cases reported and assuming a ten-day delay between infection and detection, researchers at Northeastern University estimated that the number of actual infections may be much higher than those confirmed at the time of reporting. Northeastern University estimated 21,300 infections by 26 January, increasing to 31,200 infections by 29 January (95% confidence interval 23,400–40,400). On 31

January 2020, an article in *The Lancet* estimated that 75,815 individuals (95% confidence interval 37,304–130,330) had been infected in Wuhan as of 25 January, with an estimated doubling time of 6.4 days in the period of study.

There are concerns about whether adequate medical personnel and equipment are available in regions affected by the outbreak for hospitals to correctly identify coronavirus cases instead of misdiagnosing suspected cases as "severe pneumonia". Many of those experiencing symptoms were told to self-quarantine at home instead of going to a hospital to avoid close contact with other patients with different levels of symptoms. After two repatriation flights were conducted from Wuhan to Japan in late January, 5 out of approximately 400 persons repatriated were diagnosed with the virus, of whom 1 was symptomatic, and 4 were not.

On 4 February the University of Southampton's WorldPop research group used mobile phone data and airline flight records to create a risk map for the likely spread of the disease.

Case and death counts in China are influenced by changes in clinical case definition. A paper submitted to Eurosurveillance modelling China's official death rate statistics reported that "In the popular press, there are also speculations about a large number of unreported cases, casting doubt on the usefulness of the reported numbers. Although this is justified in view of the length of the incubation period of about 6 days in this case, it affects all data uniformly.

Signs and symptoms

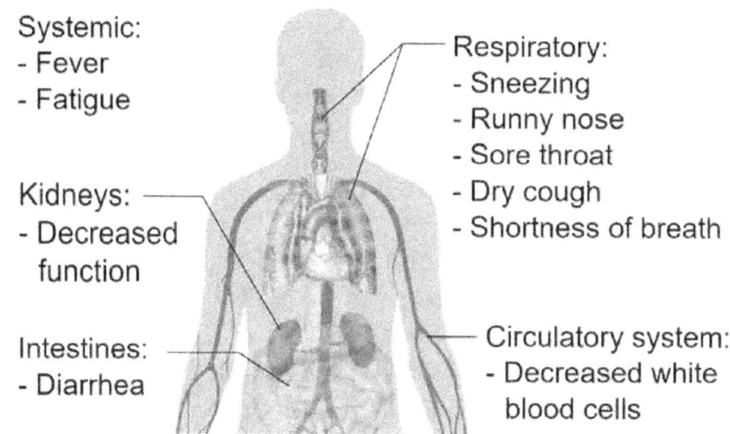

Fig. Symptoms of coronavirus disease 2019

Those infected may be asymptomatic or have mild to severe symptoms, including fever, cough, shortness of breath, and diarrhoea. The time from exposure to onset of symptoms is estimated at 2 to 10 days by WHO, and 2 to 14 days by the US Centers for Disease Control and Prevention (CDC). One study found the usual incubation time was three days but may be as long as 24 days. Upper respiratory symptoms, such as sneezing, a runny nose, and sore throat, are less frequent.

Cases of severe infection can result in pneumonia, kidney failure, and death. Among 137 early cases that were admitted to hospitals in Hubei province, 16 (12%) individuals died. Many of those who died had other conditions such as hypertension, diabetes, or cardiovascular disease that impaired their immune systems. As of 23 February 2020, the number of severe cases is 11,569 (14.7%) out of 79,364 with 24,974 having recovered.

Cause

SARS-CoV-2, a novel severe acute respiratory syndrome coronavirus first isolated from three patients with pneumonia connected to the cluster of acute respiratory illness cases reported by health authorities in Wuhan, is the causative agent of Coronavirus disease 2019 (COVID-19).

Virology

SARS-CoV-2 is closely related to SARS-Cov-1 (75% to 80% identical). It is thought to have a zoonotic origin due to its epidemiological links to the Huanan Seafood Market. Genetic analysis has revealed that the coronavirus genetically clusters with the genus Betacoronavirus, in lineage B of the subgenus Sarbecovirus together with two bat-derived strains. It is 96% identical at the whole genome level to other bat coronavirus samples. In February 2020, researchers from South China Agricultural University announced that there is a 99% similarity in genome sequences between the viruses found in pangolins and those from human patients, suggesting that the animal may be an intermediary host for the virus, but did not release evidence. At least five genomes of the novel coronavirus have been isolated and reported.

The coronavirus enters human cells through a receptor called angiotensin-converting enzyme 2 (ACE 2), a membrane exopeptidase. Bayesian analysis by Benvenuto et al. of the genome sequences of SARS-CoV-2 and related coronaviruses, shows that the nucleocapsid and the spike glycoprotein have some sites under positive selective pressure. Homology modelling indicated certain molecular and structural differences among the viruses. The phylogenetic tree showed that SARS-CoV-2 significantly clustered with a bat SARS-like coronavirus sequence, whereas structural analysis revealed mutations in spike glycoprotein and nucleocapsid protein. The authors conclude SARS-CoV-2 is a coronavirus distinct from SARS virus that probably was transmitted from bats or another host that provided the ability to infect humans.

Spread

Coronaviruses are spread through aerosol droplets expelled when an infected individual coughs or sneezes within a range of about 6 feet (1.83 m), which can contaminate surfaces like door handles or railings. Coronavirus droplets only stay suspended in the air for a short time, but can stay viable and contagious on a metal, glass or plastic surface for up to nine days. Disinfection of surfaces is possible with cheap substances such as 62–71% ethanol applied for one minute. Chinese public health officials suggest extra caution for aerosol transmission in closed rooms and recommend regularly exchanging air.

On 13 February 2020 the director of the Centers for Disease Control and Prevention of the United States confirmed asymptomatic transmission. Viral RNA was detected in stool specimens collected from the first confirmed case in the United States, though it was unclear if enough of the infectious virus was present to suggest fecal-oral transmission.

Of the initial 41 cases, two-thirds had a history of exposure to the Huanan Seafood Wholesale Market. There have been estimates for the basic reproduction number (the average number of people an infected person is likely to infect), ranging from 2.13 to 3.11. The virus has reportedly been able to transmit down a chain of up to four people so far. This is similar to severe acute respiratory syndrome-related coronavirus (SARS-CoV). There are disputed reports that some of the infected may be super-spreaders.

DIAGNOSIS

The WHO has published several testing protocols for SARS-CoV-2. Testing uses real time reverse transcription polymerase chain reaction (rRT-PCR). The test can be done on respiratory or blood samples. Results are generally available within a few hours to days.

Chinese scientists were able to isolate a strain of the coronavirus and publish the genetic sequence so that laboratories across the world could independently develop PCR tests to detect infection by the virus.

PREVENTION

There are no vaccines against SARS-CoV-2 as of 22 February 2020. Infection is primarily through human-to-human transmission, via respiratory droplets that people exhale (sneeze and cough). Though the virus is thought to have a zoonotic origin, there is no evidence that pets such as dogs and cats can be infected. The Government of Hong Kong warned anyone travelling outside the city to not touch animals; to not eat game meat; and to avoid visiting wet markets, live poultry markets, and farms.

The Ministry of Health in Singapore advises people that "those who are unwell should wear a mask and see a doctor immediately [...] but there is no need to wear a mask if you are well". It has advised against all non-essential travel to Mainland China. In addition, it lists several precautions under its health advisory:

- Do not eat raw or undercooked meats;
- Stay clear of crowded places and avoid close contact with people who are sick (something known as *social distancing*);
- Maintain good hygiene and frequently wash hands when appropriate;
- Cough or sneeze into a tissue and directly dispose of the tissue into a garbage can;
- Wear a surgical face mask if you are coughing, sneezing or have other respiratory symptoms;
- Seek prompt medical attention if you are feeling unwell.

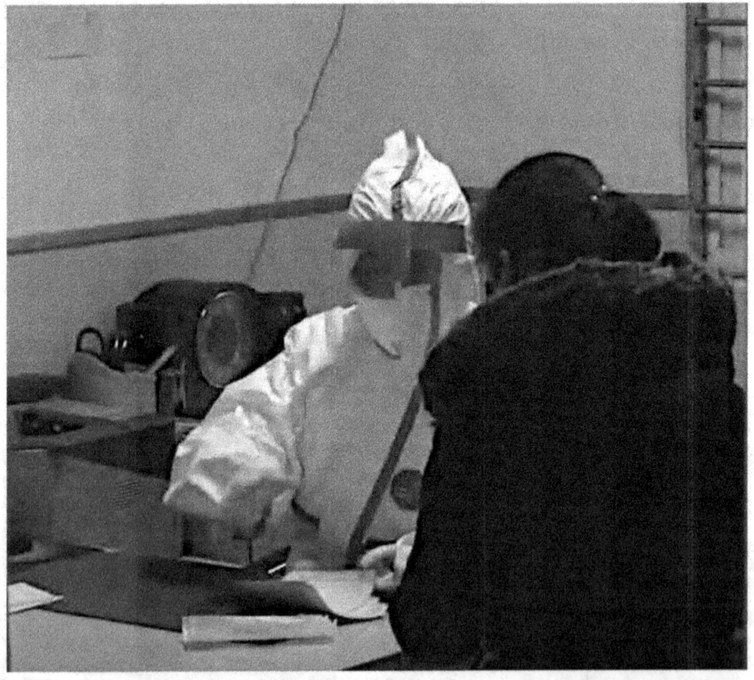

Fig. A medical worker wearing a bunny suit sees a patient in a Wuhan hospital

If a person is suspected to be infected, to prevent transmission, the U.S. CDC recommends that the infected individual stay at home except to get medical care; call ahead before visiting a healthcare provider; wear a surgical face mask (especially in public); cover coughs and sneezes with a tissue; regularly wash hands with soap and water; and avoid sharing personal household items.

Hygiene

Hand washing is recommended to prevent the spread of coronavirus. The CDC recommends that individuals:

- "Wash hands often with soap and water for at least 20 seconds, especially after going to the bathroom; before eating; and after blowing your nose, coughing, or sneezing."

- "If soap and water are not readily available, use an alcohol-based hand sanitiser with at least 60% alcohol. Always wash hands with soap and water if hands are visibly dirty."

The CDC, NHS, and WHO also advise individuals to avoid touching the eyes, nose, or mouth with unwashed hands.

Coronaviruses can survive and remain contagious on a metal, glass or plastic surface for up to nine days. Methods to remove the virus from surfaces include chlorine-based disinfectants, 75% ethanol, peracetic acid, and chloroform.

Respiratory hygiene

Those who suspect they are infected should wear a surgical mask (especially when in public) and call a doctor for medical advice. By limiting the volume and travel distance of expiratory droplets dispersed when talking, sneezing, and coughing, masks can serve a public health benefit in reducing transmission by those unknowingly infected.

If a mask is not available, anyone experiencing respiratory symptoms should cover a cough or sneeze with a tissue, promptly discard it in the trash, and wash their hands. If a tissue is unavailable, individuals can cover their mouth or nose with a flexed elbow.

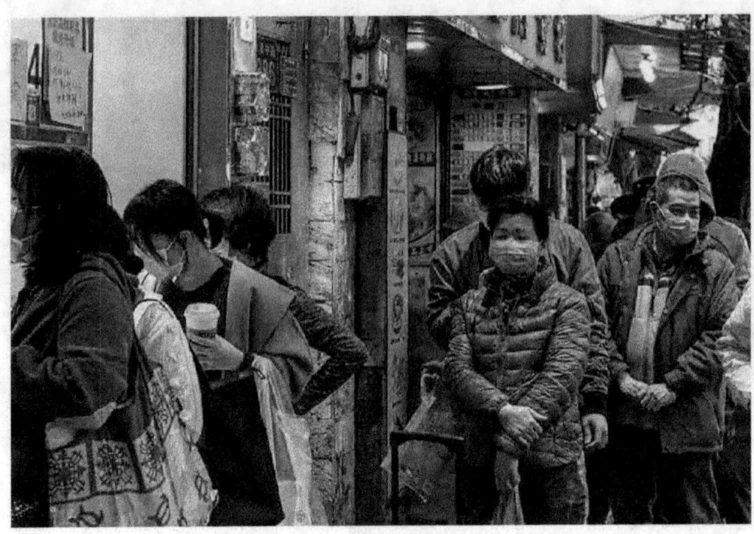

Surgical masks used by people in Guangzhou. Masks are not recommended for people at low risk of infection.

Masks are also recommended for those taking care of someone who may have the disease. Rinsing the nose, gargling with mouthwash, and eating garlic are not effective.

There is no evidence to show that masks protect uninfected persons at low risk and wearing them may create a false sense of security.

Surgical masks are widely used by healthy people in Hong Kong, Japan, Singapore and Malaysia. Surgical masks are not recommended by the CDC as a preventive measure for the American general public.

The WHO advises the following best practices for mask usage:

- Place mask carefully to cover mouth and nose and tie securely to minimise any gaps between the face and the mask; While in use, avoid touching the mask;
- Remove the mask by using appropriate technique (i.e. do not touch the front but remove the lace from behind);
- After removal or whenever you inadvertently touch a used mask, clean hands by using an alcohol-based hand rub or soap and water if visibly soiled
- Replace masks with a new clean, dry mask as soon as they become damp/humid;
- Do not re-use single-use masks; Discard single-use masks after each use and dispose of them immediately upon removal

Healthcare professionals interacting directly with people who have the disease are advised to use respirators at least as protective as NIOSH-certified N95, EU standard FFP2, or equivalent, in addition to other personal protective equipment.

Vaccine and therapy research

Several organisations around the world are developing vaccines or testing antiviral medicine. In China, the Chinese Center for Disease Control and Prevention (CCDC) has started developing vaccines against the novel coronavirus and is testing existing drug effectiveness for pneumonia. Also, a team at the University of Hong Kong announced that a new vaccine is developed, but needs to be tested on animals before conducting clinical tests on humans.

In Western countries, the United States' National Institutes of Health (NIH) is hoping for human trials of a vaccine by April 2020; the Norwegian Coalition for Epidemic Preparedness Innovations (CEPI) is funding three vaccine projects and hopes to have a vaccine in trials by June 2020, and approved and ready in a year. These projects are an mRNA vaccine developed by Cambridge, Massachusetts–based Moderna, a "molecular clamp" vaccine platform the University of Queensland in Australia is developing after receiving AU$10.6 million in funding from CEPI, and a vaccine Inovio Pharmaceuticals designed in two hours after receiving the gene sequence of the virus. The latter vaccine is being manufactured so that it can be first tested on animals. By February 2020, United States Department of Health and Human Services' Biomedical Advanced Research and Development Authority announced partnerships with Johnson & Johnson's Janssen Pharmaceutica and Sanofi Pasteur to develop vaccines and to screen for potential drugs in collaboration with the Belgium-based Rega Institute for Medical Research.

Management

Infrared cameras were installed in Wuhan railway station to check passengers' body temperature before they board the trains.

There are no specific medications for SARS-CoV-2, though development efforts are underway. Attempts to relieve the symptoms include taking regular (over-the-counter) flu medications, drinking fluids, and resting. Depending on the severity, oxygen therapy, intravenous fluids, and breathing support may be required. Some countries require people to report flu-like symptoms to their doctor, especially if they have visited mainland China.

On 18 February 2020, the Chinese National Medical Products Administration approved the antiviral drug Favilavir (formerly Fapinavir) for use against COVID-19. The drug, previously approved for treatment of influenza, had shown early efficacy against COVID-19 in human trials in China.

Domestic responses

The first person known to have fallen ill due to the new virus was in Wuhan on 1 December 2019. A public notice on the outbreak was released 30 days later by Wuhan health authority on 31 December 2019; the initial notice informed Wuhan residents that there was no clear evidence of human-to-human transmission of the virus, that the disease is preventable and controllable, and that people can wear masks when going out. WHO was informed of the outbreak on the same day.

On 7 January 2020, Chinese Communist Party general secretary Xi Jinping, chaired the meeting of Party Politburo Standing Committee to discuss novel coronavirus prevention and control.

On 20 January, Zhong Nanshan, a scientist at China's National Health Commission who played a prominent role in the SARS epidemic, declared its potential for human-to-human transmission, after 2 cases emerged in Guangdong province of infection by family members who had visited Wuhan. This was later confirmed by the Wuhan government, which announced a number of new measures such as cancelling the Chinese New Year celebrations, in addition to measures such as checking the temperature of passengers at transport terminals first introduced on 14 January. A quarantine was announced on 23 January 2020 stopping travel in and out of Wuhan.

On 25 January, Politburo of the Communist Party of China met to discuss novel coronavirus prevention and control. Chinese Communist Party general secretary Xi Jinping stated that the country is facing a "grave situation" as the number of infected people is accelerating. In the evening, the authorities banned the use of private vehicles in Wuhan. Only vehicles that are transporting critical supplies or emergency response vehicles are allowed to move within the city.

On 26 January, a leading group tasked with the prevention and control of the novel coronavirus outbreak was established, led by Chinese Premier Li Keqiang. Premier Li visited Wuhan to direct the epidemic prevention work on 27 January. The leading group has decided to extend Spring Festival holiday to contain coronavirus outbreak.

China Customs started requiring that all passengers entering and exiting China fill in an extra health declaration form from 26 January. The health declaration form was mentioned in China's Frontier Health and Quarantine Law, granting the customs rights to require it if needed. The customs said it will "restart this system" as it was not a requirement before.

On 27 January, the General Office of the State Council of China, one of the top governing bodies of the People's Republic, officially declared a nation-wide extension on the New Year holiday and the postponement of the coming spring semester. The

Office extended the previously scheduled public holiday from 30 January to 2 February, while it said school openings for the spring semester will be announced in the future. Some universities with open campuses also banned the public from visiting. On 23 January, the education department in Hunan, which neighbours the centre of the outbreak Hubei province, stated it will strictly ban off-school tutors and restrict student gatherings.

Education departments in Shanghai and Shenzhen also imposed bans on off-school tutoring and requested that schools track and report students who had been to Wuhan or Hubei province during the winter break. The semi-autonomous regions of Hong Kong and Macau also announced adjustments on schooling schedules. Hong Kong's Chief Executive Carrie Lam declared an emergency at a press conference on 25 January, saying the government will close primary and secondary schools for two more weeks on top of the previously scheduled New Year holiday, pushing the date for school reopening to 17 February. Macau closed several museums and libraries, and prolonged the New Year holiday break to 11 February for higher education institutions and 10 February for others. The University of Macau said they would track the physical conditions of students who have been to Wuhan during the New Year break.

After the Chinese New Year on 25 January, there would be another peak of people travelling back from their hometowns to workplaces as a part of Chunyun. Several provinces and cities encouraged people to stay in their hometowns and not travel back. Eastern China's Suzhou also encouraged remote working via the Internet and further prolonged the spring festival break.

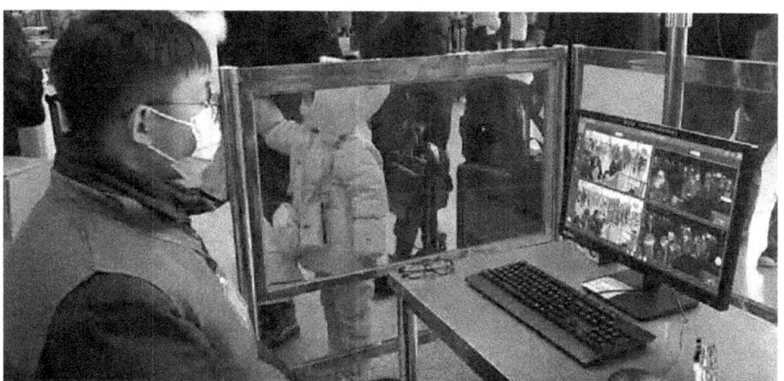

Fig. Infrared cameras were installed in Wuhan railway station to check passengers' body temperature before they board the trains.

The Civil Aviation Administration of China and the China State Railway Group, which regulates China's civil aviation and operates rail services, announced on 24 January that passengers could have full refunds for their plane and train tickets without any additional surcharges, regardless of whether their flight or train will go through Wuhan or not. Some hotel chains and online travel agencies also allowed more flexibility in cancellations and changes. China's Ministry of Culture and Tourism ordered travel agencies and online tourism firms to suspend package tours and stop offering "flight+hotel" bundles.

Additional provinces and cities outside Hubei imposed travel restrictions. Beijing suspended all intercity bus services on 25 January, with several others following suit. Shanghai, Tianjin, Shandong, Xi'an, and Sanya all announced suspension of intercity or inter-province bus services on 26 January.

On 1 February 2020, Xinhua News reported that China's Supreme People's Procuratorate (SPP) has "asked procuratorates nationwide to fully play their role to create a favourable judicial environment in the fight against the novel coronavirus outbreak." This includes severe punishments for those found guilty of dereliction of duty and the withholding of information for officials. Tougher charges were proscribed for commercial criminal activities such as "the pushing up of prices, profiteering and severely disturbing market order" along with the "production and sale of fake and shoddy protective equipment and medicines." Prosecuting actions against patients who deliberately spread the infection or refuse examination or compulsory isolation along with threats of violence against medical personnel were also urged. The statement also included urging to prosecute those found "fabricating coronavirus-related information that may lead to panic among the public, making up and spreading rumors about the virus, sabotaging the implementation of the law and endangering public security" and also stressed harsh punishment for the illegal hunting of wildlife under state protection, as well as improving inspection and quarantine measures for fresh food and meat products."

Museums throughout China are temporarily closed. To provide cultural and heritage seekers some form of service, the Chinese National Cultural Heritage Administration (NCHA) has asked museums around the country to move their exhibits and galleries temporarily online. This is done via a specific program that the NCHA is launching. Some museums are also putting the content on their own website, social media, or even social chat apps and rooms like WeChat. The majority of the content will be available on a NCHA website web page, however it is only accessible inside of China. However, there are a few excerpts from the main created exhibition website that are on the NCHA general information page that are linked too, that are accessible outside of China.

On 23 January 2020, a quarantine on travel in and out of Wuhan was imposed in an effort to stop the spread of the virus out of Wuhan. Flights, trains, public buses, the metro system, and long-distance coaches were suspended indefinitely. Large-scale gatherings and group tours were also suspended. By 24 January 2020, a total of 15 cities in Hubei, including Wuhan, were placed under similar quarantine measures. On 27 and 28 January 2020, Xiangyang closed its railway stations and suspended all ferry operations, after shutting down its airport and intercity bus services earlier. Thus, the entire Hubei province entered a city-by-city quarantine, save for the Shennongjia Forestry District.

Before the quarantine began, some in Wuhan questioned the reliability of the figures from the Chinese government as well as the government response, with some calling for quarantine, and a post also showed sick people and three dead bodies covered in white sheets on the floor of a hospital on 24 January, although many such posts in Weibo about the epidemic have since been deleted.

Due to quarantine measures, Wuhan residents rushed to stockpile essential goods, food, and fuel; prices rose significantly. 5,000,000 people left Wuhan, with 9,000,000 left in the city.

On 26 January, the city of Shantou in Guangdong declared a partial lockdown, though this was reversed two hours later. Residents had rushed to supermarkets to stock food as soon as the lockdown was declared, until the authorities reversed their decision. *Caixin* said, that the wording of Shantou's initial declaration was "unprecedentedly strict" and will severely affect residents' lives, if implemented as-is. Shantou's Department for Outbreak Control later clarified, that they will not restrict travelling, and all they would do, is to sterilise vehicles used for transportation.

Local authorities in Beijing and several other major cities, including Hangzhou, Guangzhou, Shanghai, and Shenzhen, announced on 26 January, that these cities will not impose a lockdown similar to those in Hubei province. Rumours of these potential lockdowns had spread widely prior to the official announcements. A spokesperson of Beijing's Municipal Transportation Commission claimed, that the expressways and highways, as well as subways and buses were operating normally. To ease the residents' panic, the Hangzhou city government stressed that the city would not be locked down from the outside world, and both cities said that they would introduce precautions against potential risks.

On 2 February 2020, the city of Wenzhou in Zhejiang province also implemented a partial lockdown, closing 46 of the 54 highway checkpoints.

On 4 February 2020, two more cities in Zhejiang province restricted the movement of residents. The city of Taizhou, three Hangzhou districts, and some in Ningbo began to only allow one person per household to go outside every two days to buy necessities, city officials said. More than 12 million people are affected by the new restrictions.

By 6 February 2020, a total of four Zhejiang cities—Wenzhou, Hangzhou, Ningbo, and Taizhou—were under the "passport" system, allowing only one person per household to leave their home every two days. These restrictions apply to over 30 million people.

Outside Mainland China, some cruise ships were quarantined after passengers developed symptoms or tested positive for SARS-CoV-2. The *Costa Smeralda* was quarantined on 30 January off Civitavecchia in Italy, after passengers developed flu-like symptoms – the quarantine was lifted when tests for the virus came back negative. Two further ships were quarantined on 5 February: *Diamond Princess* in the Port of Yokohama, Japan and *World Dream*, which returned to Hong Kong after being refused entry to Kaohsiung, Taiwan. In both cases, passengers and crew tested positive. On 10 February passengers were allowed to disembark the *World Dream* "without the need to self-quarantine after leaving." The *Diamond Princess* remains quarantined with 136 confirmed cases as of 10 February. Although the quarantine has not been completely lifted, around 500 passengers that were not diagnosed with the virus were allowed to leave on 19 February 2020. In addition, although not quarantined the MS Westerdam has been refused entry by several ports after departing Hong Kong on 1 February.

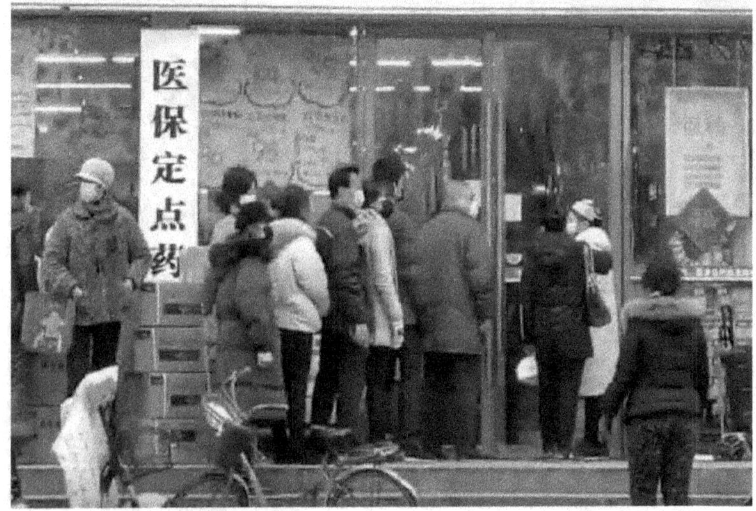

People queueing outside a Wuhan pharmacy to buy face masks and medical supplies

Outdoor restrictions

On 1 February, Huanggang, Hubei implemented a measure whereby only one person from each household is permitted to go outside for provisions once every two days, except for medical reasons or to work at shops or pharmacies. Many cities, districts, and counties across mainland China implemented similar measures in the days following, including Wenzhou, Hangzhou, Fuzhou, Harbin, and the whole of Jiangxi Province.

Censorship and police responses

The first known infection by a new virus was reported in Wuhan on 1 December 2019. The early response by city authorities was accused of prioritising a control of information on the outbreak. A group of eight medical personnel, including Li Wenliang, an ophthalmologist from Wuhan Central Hospital, who in late December posted warnings on a new coronavirus strain akin to SARS, were warned by Wuhan police for "spreading rumours" for likening it to SARS.

By the time China had informed the World Health Organization of the new coronavirus on 31 December 2019, the *New York Times* reported that the government was still keeping "its own citizens in the dark". While by a number of measures, China's initial handling of the crisis was an improvement in relation to the SARS response in 2003, China has been criticised for cover-ups and downplaying the initial discovery and severity of the outbreak. This has been attributed to the censorship institutional structure of the country's press and internet, with the *New York Times* Nicholas Kristof and CSIS's Jude Blanchette suggesting that it was exacerbated by China's paramount leader Xi Jinping's crackdown on independent oversight such as journalism and social media that left senior officials with inaccurate information on the outbreak and "contributed to a prolonged period of inaction that allowed the virus to spread".

On 20 January, General Secretary Xi Jinping made his first public remark on the outbreak and spoke of "the need for the timely release of information". Chinese premier Li Keqiang also urged efforts to prevent and control the epidemic. One day later, the CPC Central Political and Legal Affairs Commission, the most powerful political organ in China overseeing legal enforcement and the police, wrote "self-deception will only make the epidemic worse and turn a natural disaster that was controllable into a man-made disaster at great cost," and "only openness can minimise panic to the greatest extent." The commission then added, "anyone who deliberately delays and hides the reporting of cases out of self-interest will be nailed on a pillar of shame for eternity." Also on the same day, Xi Jinping instructed authorities "to strengthen the guidance of public opinions", language which some view as a call for censorship after commentators on social media became increasingly pointedly critical and angry at the government due to the epidemic. Some view this as contradictory to the calls for "openness" that the central government had already declared.

Statements issued by Xi Jinping on 3 February declared the need for an emphasis by state media on "telling the moving stories of how [people] on the front line are preventing and fighting the virus" as a priority of coverage, while top official Zhang Xiaoguo said that his department would "treat propaganda regarding the control and prevention measures of the virus as its top priority". The Cyberspace Administration (CAC) declared its intent to foster an "good online atmosphere," with CAC notices sent to video platforms encouraging them to "not to push any negative story, and not to conduct non-official livestreaming on the virus."

Censorship has been observed being applied on news articles and social media posts deemed to hold negative tones about the coronavirus and the governmental response, including posts mocking Xi Jinping for not visiting areas of the epidemic, an article that predicted negative effects of the epidemic on the economy, and calls to remove local government officials. Chinese citizens have reportedly used innovative methods to avoid censorship to express anger about how government officials have handled the initial outbreak response, such as using the word 'Trump' to refer to Xi Jinping, or 'Chernobyl' to refer to the outbreak as a whole. While censorship had been briefly relaxed giving a "window of about two weeks in which Chinese journalists were able to publish hard-hitting stories exposing the mishandling of the novel coronavirus by officials", since then private news outlets were reportedly required to use "planned and controlled publicity" with the authorities' consent.

On 30 January, China's Supreme Court, delivered a rare rebuke against the country's police forces, calling the "unreasonably harsh crackdown on online rumours" as undermining public trust. In what has been called a "highly unusual criticism" by observers, supreme court judge Tang Xinghua said that if police had been lenient against rumours and allowed the public to have taken heed of them, an earlier adoption of "measures like wearing masks, strictly disinfecting and avoiding wildlife markets" might have been useful in countering the spread of the epidemic. The Human Rights Watch reported that "there is considerable misinformation on Chinese social media and authorities have legitimate reasons to counter false information that can cause public panic," but also noted censorship by the authorities on social media posted by families of infected people who were potentially seeking help as well as by people living in cordoned cities who were documenting their daily lives amidst the lockdown.

After the death of Li Wenliang, who was widely hailed as a whistleblower in China on 7 February, some of the trending hashtags on Weibo such as "Wuhan government owes Dr Li Wenliang an apology" and "We want freedom of speech" were blocked. While media outlets were allowed to report his death, the nature of the doctor's censorship which produced widespread public anger in the aftermath, in what has been described as "one of the biggest outpourings of online criticism of the government in years," was not a topic that was permitted for coverage. One such media outlet even sending notices to editors, and leaked to reporters, asking them to refrain from "commenting or speculating" and giving instructions to "not hashtag and let the topic gradually die out from the hot search list, and guard against harmful information." After attempts to discourage the discussion on Dr. Li's death further escalated online anger, the central government has reportedly attempted to reshape the narrative by "cast[ing] Dr. Li's death as the nation's sacrifice — meaning, the Chinese Communist Party's own". A group of Chinese academics including Xu Zhangrun of Tsinghua University signed an open letter calling for the central government to issue an apology to Dr. Li and to protect freedom of speech. Professor Zhou Lian of Renmin University has observed that the epidemic has "allowed more people to see the institutional factors behind the outbreak and the importance of freedom of speech".

International responses

Since 31 December 2019, some regions and countries near China tightened their screening of selected travellers. The Centers for Disease Control and Prevention (CDC) of the United States later issued a Level 1 travel watch. Guidances and risk assessments were shortly posted by others including the European Centre for Disease Prevention and Control and Public Health England. In China, airports, railway stations and coach stations installed infrared thermometers. Travellers with a measured fever are taken to medical institutions after being registered and given masks. Real time Reverse Transcription-Polymerase Chain Reaction (rRT-PCR) test was used to confirm new cases of coronavirus infection.

An analysis of air travel patterns was used to map out and predict patterns of spread and was published in the *Journal of Travel Medicine* in mid-January 2020. Based on information from the International Air Transport Association (2018), Bangkok, Hong Kong, Tokyo, and Taipei had the largest volume of travellers from Wuhan. Dubai, Sydney and Melbourne were also reported as popular destinations for people travelling from Wuhan. Using the validated tool, the Infectious Disease Vulnerability Index (IDVI), to assess the ability to manage a disease threat, Bali was reported as least able in preparedness, while cities in Australia were considered most able.

As a result of the outbreak many countries including most of the Schengen area, Armenia, Australia, India, Iraq, Indonesia, Kazakhstan, Kuwait, Malaysia, Maldives, Mongolia, New Zealand, Philippines, Singapore, Sri Lanka, Taiwan, Vietnam, and the United States have imposed temporary entry bans on Chinese citizens or recent visitors to China, or have ceased issuing visas and reimposed visa requirements on Chinese citizens. Samoa even started refusing entry to its own citizens who had previously been to China, attracting widespread condemnation over the legality of such decision.

In Asia, Hong Kong, Mongolia, Nepal, North Korea, Russia, and Vietnam have also responded with border tightening/closures with mainland China. On 22 January 2020, North Korea closed its borders to international tourists to prevent the spread of the virus into the country. Chinese visitors make up the bulk of foreign tourists to North Korea.

Also on 22 January, the Asian Football Confederation (AFC) announced that it would be moving the matches in the third round of the 2020 AFC Women's Olympic Qualifying Tournament from Wuhan to Nanjing, affecting the women's national team squads from Australia, China PR, Chinese Taipei, and Thailand. A few days later, the AFC announced that together with Football Federation Australia they would be moving the matches to Sydney. The Asia-Pacific Olympic boxing qualifiers, which were originally set to be held in Wuhan from 3–14 February, were also cancelled and moved to Amman, Jordan to be held between 3–11 March.

On 27 January 2020, the United States CDC issued updated travel guidance for China, recommending that travellers avoid all nonessential travel to all of the country. The CDC has directed US Customs and Border Protection to check individuals for symptoms of the coronavirus.

On 29 January 2020, British Airways, Lufthansa, Lion Air, and Air Seoul cancelled all their flights to mainland China in reaction to the spread of the virus. The same day, the Czech Republic stopped issuing Schengen visas to Chinese citizens. On 30 January 2020, Belgium, Greece and Italy closed all Schengen Visa application centres in China. The same day, Egyptair announced suspension of flights between Egypt and Hangzhou starting 1 February 2020 while those to Beijing and Guangzhou will be suspended starting 4 February 2020 until further notice.

On 31 January 2020, Italy suspended all passenger air traffic to Italy from Mainland China, Hong Kong, Macau, and Taiwan. The Italian Civil Aviation Authority NOTAM says that effective 31 January, all passenger flights from China, including the special administrative regions of Hong Kong and Macau, and Taiwan are suspended until further notice, on request of the Italian health authorities. Aircraft that were flying to Italy when the NOTAM was published, were cleared to land.

As of 1 February 2020, France was the only remaining Schengen country still issuing visas to Chinese citizens.

Qatar Airways took the decision to suspend flights to mainland China from 3 February until further notice, due to significant operational challenges caused by entry restrictions imposed by several countries. Qatar Airways is the first carrier in the Middle East to do so. An ongoing review of operations will be conducted weekly with the intention to reinstate flights as soon as the restrictions are lifted.

Though some of the airlines cancelled flights to Hong Kong as well, British Airways, Finnair and Lufthansa have not, and American Airlines continues operating a limited service to the area. Hong Kong's four airlines halved the flights to mainland China. A large number of airlines have reduced or cancelled flights to and from China. On 31 January 2020, the United States declared the virus a public health emergency. Starting 2 February, all inbound passengers who have been to Hubei in the previous 14 days will be put under quarantine for up to 14 days. Any US citizen who has travelled to the rest of mainland China will be allowed to continue their travel home if they are asymptomatic, but will be monitored by local health departments.

On 2 February 2020, India issued a travel advisory that warned all people residing in India to not travel to China, suspended E-visas from China, and further stated anyone who has travelled to China starting 15 January (to an indefinite point in the future) could be quarantined. New Zealand announced that it will deny entry to all travellers from China and that it will order its citizens to self-isolate for 14 days if they are returning from China. Indonesia and Iraq followed by also banning all travellers that visited China within the past 14 days.

On 3 February 2020, Indonesia announced it would ban passenger flights and also sea freight from and to China starting on 5 February and until further notice. Live animal imports and other products were banned as well. Minister of Trade Agus Suparmanto "We will obviously stop live animals imports from China and are still considering banning other products" Turkey announced it would suspend all flights from China till the end of February and begin scanning passengers coming from South Asian countries at airports.

Australia released its Australian Health Sector Emergency Response Plan for Novel Coronavirus (COVID-19) in February 07, 2020. It states that, although much is yet to be known about COVID-19, "Australia has taken a precautionary approach in line with preparedness and response guidance for a pandemic, working collaboratively with state and territory and whole of government partners to implement strategies to minimise disease transmission through strong border measures and widespread communication activities."

Evacuation of Foreign Citizens

Due to the effective lockdown of public transport in Wuhan and Hubei, several countries have planned to evacuate their citizens and diplomatic staff from the area, primarily through chartered flights of the home nation that have been provided clearance by Chinese authorities. Canada, the United States, Japan, India, France, Australia, Sri Lanka, Germany and Thailand were among the first to plan the evacuation of their citizens. Pakistan has said that it will not be evacuating any citizens from China.

On 7 February, Brazil evacuated 34 Brazilians or family members in addition to four Poles, a Chinese and an Indian citizen. The citizens of Poland, China and India got off the plane in Poland, where the Brazilian plane made a stopover before following its route to Brazil. Brazilian citizens who went to Brazil were quarantined at a military base near Brasilia.

On 7 February 215 Canadians (176 from the first plane, and 39 from a second plane chartered by the U.S. government) were evacuated from Wuhan, China, to CFB Trenton to be quarantined for two weeks. On 11 February, another plane of Canadians (185) from Wuhan landed at CFB Trenton. Australian authorities evacuated 277 citizens on 3 and 4 February to the Christmas Island Detention Centre which had been "repurposed" as a quarantine facility, where they remained for 14 days. United States announced that it will evacuate Americans currently aboard the cruise ship Diamond Princess. On 21 February, a plane carrying 129 Canadian passengers evacuated from the Diamond Princess landed in Trenton, Ontario.

International aid

On 5 February, the Chinese foreign ministry stated that 21 countries (including Belarus, Pakistan, Trinidad and Tobago, Egypt, and Iran) had sent aid to China.

The United States city of Pittsburgh announced plans to promptly send aid to Wuhan, with mayor Bill Peduto stating that "Our office has reached out to the mayor of Wuhan, which is our sister city" and promising that "over the next two days we should be able to have a care package that has been put together." He speculated that the contents of such a package will be coordinated with the consultation of medical experts, but that it will likely consist of "face masks, rubber gloves and other material that could be hard to find in the future".

Additionally, the University of Pittsburgh Medical Center (UPMC) announced plans to provide help, with UPMC spokesman Paul Wood stating that "UPMC has a significant presence in China and has been in contact with our partners there", also declaring that "we stand ready to assist them and others in China with their unmet humanitarian needs." Some Chinese students at other American universities have also joined together to help send aid to virus-stricken parts of China, with a joint group in the Greater Chicago Area reportedly managing to send 50,000 N95 masks and 1,500 protection suits to hospitals in the Hubei province on 30 January.

The humanitarian aid organisation Direct Relief, in co-ordination with FedEx transportation and logistics support, sent 200,000 face masks along with other personal protective equipment, including gloves and gowns, by emergency airlift to arrive in Wuhan Union Hospital, who requested the supplies by 30 January. The Gates Foundation stated on 26 January that it would donate US$5 million in aid to support the response in China that will be aimed at assisting "emergency funds and corresponding technical support to help front-line responders". On 5 February, Bill and Melinda further announced a $100 million donation to the World Health Organization, who made an appeal for funding contributions to the international community the same day. The donation will be used to fund vaccine research and treatment efforts along with protecting "at-risk populations in Africa and South Asia."

Japan, in the process of co-ordinating a plane flight to Wuhan to pick up Japanese nationals in the city, has promised that the plane will first carry into Wuhan aid supplies that Japanese foreign minister Toshimitsu Motegi stated will consist of "masks and protective suits for Chinese people as well as for Japanese nationals". On 26 January, the plane arrived in Wuhan, donating its supply of one million face masks to the city. Also among the aid supplies were 20,000 protective suits for medical staff across Hubei donated by the Tokyo Metropolitan Government.

Support efforts have sprung across Japan to help aid residents in Wuhan. On 27 January, the city of Ôita, a sister city to Wuhan for 40 years, sent 30,000 masks from its own disaster relief stockpile to its sister city through the Red Cross network with boxes labelled "Wuhan Jiayou!", meaning "Hang in there, Wuhan!" in Chinese. Its International Affairs Office division head, Soichiro Hayashi, said that "The people of Wuhan are like family" and expressed hopes that "people can return to their ordinary lives as quickly as possible".

On 28 January, the city of Mito donated 50,000 masks to its sister-city of Chongqing, and on 6 February, the city of Okayama sent 22,000 masks to Luoyang, its own sister-city. The ruling Liberal Democratic Party on 10 February made a symbolic deduction of 5,000 yen from the March salary of every LDP parliamentarian, a total of 2 million yen, to donate to China, with the party's secretary-general, Toshihiro Nikai, stating that "For Japan, when it sees a virus outbreak in China, it is like seeing a relative or neighbour suffering. Japanese people are willing to help China and hope the outbreak will pass as soon as possible."

Peace Winds Japan has declared it will send a staff member to China to help distribute the face masks and other goods that the NGO will send to the country.

A number of other countries have also announced aid efforts. Malaysia announced a donation of 18 million medical gloves to China, The Philippine Red Cross also donated $1.4 million worth of Philippine-made face masks, which were shipped to Wuhan. Turkey dispatched medical equipment, and Germany delivered various medical supplies including 10,000 Hazmat suits. On 19 February, Singapore Red Cross announced that they will send $2.26 million worth of aid to China, which they declared would consist of "purchasing and distributing protective equipment like surgical masks for hospital staff and other healthcare workers." It will also be used to "buy and distribute hygiene items and conduct health education in seven welfare homes in Tianjin and Nanning."

Speciality hospitals

A speciality hospital named Huoshenshan Hospital has been constructed as a countermeasure against the outbreak and to better quarantine the patients. Wuhan City government had demanded that a state-owned enterprise construct such a hospital "at the fastest speed" comparable to that of the SARS outbreak in 2003. On 24 January, Wuhan authorities specified its planning, saying they planned to have Huoshenshan Hospital built within six days of the announcement and it will be ready to use on 3 February. Upon opening, the speciality hospital has 1,000 beds and takes up 30,000 square metres. The hospital is modelled after the Xiaotangshan Hospital [zh], which was fabricated for the SARS outbreak of 2003, itself built in only seven days. State media reported that there were 7,000 workers and nearly 300 units of construction machinery on the site at peak.

On 25 January authorities announced plans for Leishenshan Hospital, a second speciality hospital, with a capacity of 1,600 beds; operations are scheduled to start by 6 February. Some people voiced their concerns through social media services, saying the authorities' decision to build yet another hospital in such little time showed the severity of the outbreak could be a lot worse than expected.

On 24 January 2020, the authority announced that they would convert an empty building in Huangzhou District, Huanggang to a 1,000-bed hospital named Dabie Mountain Regional Medical Centre. Works began the next day by 500 personnel and the building began accepting patients on 28 January 2020 at 10:30 pm. In Wuhan, authorities have seized dormitories, offices and hospitals to create more beds for patients.

REACTIONS TO PREVENTION EFFORTS

WHO response measures

The World Health Organization (WHO) has commended the efforts of Chinese authorities in managing and containing the epidemic, with Director-General Tedros

Adhanom Ghebreyesus expressing "confidence in China's approach to controlling the epidemic" and calling for the public to "remain calm". The WHO noted the contrast between the 2003 epidemic, where Chinese authorities were accused of secrecy that impeded prevention and containment efforts, and the current crisis where the central government "has provided regular updates to avoid panic ahead of Lunar New Year holidays".

The WHO and Chinese authorities have also received criticism for their delayed reporting and handling of the epidemic, leading to scrutiny of the relationship between the two entities amid allegations of a cover-up. The WHO relies upon data provided and filtered by member states, with China have a "historical aversion to transparency and sensitivity to international criticism". John Mackenzie of the WHO's emergency committee and Anne Schuchat of the Centers for Disease Control and Prevention in Washington suggested that China's official tally of cases and deaths was an underestimation. Others noted that China lumped Taiwan with the semi-autonomous regions of Hong Kong and Macao when reporting outbreak data, resulting in Taiwan receiving the same WHO "very high" risk rating as the mainland despite only a small number of cases on the self-governing island. Insiders at the US Centres for Disease Control and Prevention complained that China would not agree to on-site visits, while it took two weeks for Chinese authorities to approve an international mission team led by Dr. Bruce Aylward but the team composition and scope of work was still yet to be determined. Taiwan, which has long been excluded from the WHO for refusing to adhere to the "One China" policy, was only granted participation for this outbreak after "lobbying by countries including the U.S."

In response to the criticisms, Tedros stated that China "doesn't need to be asked to be praised. China has done many good things to slow down the virus. The whole world can judge. There is no spinning here."

Some attacked Tedros for his apparent appeasement to avoid "antagoniz[ing] the notoriously touchy Chinese government even though it is clear the country has been less than fully transparent about the outbreak's early stages, and perhaps still is". Others including Dr. David Nabarro have defended this strategy in order "to ensure Beijing's co-operation in mounting an effective global response to the outbreak".

In reaction to the central authorities' decision to implement a transportation ban in Wuhan, WHO representative Gauden Galea remarked that while it was "certainly not a recommendation the WHO has made", it was also "a very important indication of the commitment to contain the epidemic in the place where it is most concentrated" and called it "unprecedented in public health history". Unlike the recommendations of other agencies, Tedros stated that "there is no reason for measures that unnecessarily interfere with international travel and trade" and that "WHO doesn't recommend limiting trade and movement".

On 30 January 2020, following confirmation of human-to-human transmission outside China and the increase in number of cases in other countries, the WHO declared the outbreak a Public Health Emergency of International Concern (PHEIC), the sixth PHEIC since the measure was first invoked during the 2009 swine flu pandemic. Tedros clarified that the PHEIC, in this case, was "not a vote of no confidence in China", but because of the risk of global spread, especially to low- and middle-income countries without robust health systems.

On 5 February, the WHO appealed to the global community for a $675 million contribution to fund strategic preparedness in low-income countries, citing the urgency to develop those countries which "do not have the systems in place to detect people who have contracted the virus, even if it were to emerge." Tedros further made statements declaring that "We are only as strong as our weakest link" and urged the international community to "invest today or pay more later."

On 11 February, the WHO in a press conference established COVID-19 as the name of the disease. In a further statement on the same day, Tedros stated that he had briefed with UN Secretary General Antonio Guterres who agreed to provide the "power of the entire UN system in the response." A UN Crisis Management Team was activated as a result, allowing co-ordination of the entire United Nations response, which the WHO states will allow them to "focus on the health response while the other agencies can bring their expertise to bear on the wider social, economic and developmental implications of the outbreak."

On 14 February, a WHO-led Joint Mission Team with China was activated to provide international and WHO experts to touch ground in China to assist in the domestic management and evaluate "the severity and the transmissibility of the disease" by hosting workshops and meetings with key national-level institutions to conduct field visits to assess the "impact of response activities at provincial and county levels, including urban and rural settings."

International reactions

China's response to the virus, in comparison to the 2003 SARS outbreak, has been praised by some foreign leaders. US president Donald Trump thanked Chinese President Xi Jinping "on behalf of the American People" on 24 January 2020 on Twitter, stating that "China has been working very hard to contain the Coronavirus. The United States greatly appreciates their efforts and transparency" and declaring that "It will all work out well." Germany's health minister Jens Spahn, in an interview on Bloomberg TV, said with comparison to the Chinese response to SARS in 2003: "There's a big difference to SARS. We have a much more transparent China. The action of China is much more effective in the first days already." He also praised the international co-operation and communication in dealing with the virus.

At a Sunday mass at St. Peter's Square in Vatican City on 26 January 2020, Pope Francis praised "the great commitment by the Chinese community that has already been put in place to combat the epidemic" and commenced a closing prayer for "the people who are sick because of the virus that has spread through China".

Criticism of responses

Wuhan and Hubei government

Local officials in Wuhan and the province of Hubei have faced criticism, both domestically and internationally, for mishandling the initial outbreak. Allegations included insufficient medical supplies, lack of transparency to the press and censorship of social media during the initial weeks of the outbreak. On 1 January 2020, the Wuhan police interviewed eight residents for "spreading false information" (characterising the new infection as SARS-like). The Wuhan police had originally stated through a post on its official Weibo account that "eight people had been dealt with according to the law", later clarifying through Weibo that they had only given out "education and criticism" and refrained from harsher punishments such as "warnings, fines, or detention". One of the eight, a doctor named Li Wenliang who informed his former medical school classmates of the coronavirus in a WeChat group after examining a patient's medical report with symptoms of the illness, was warned by the police on 3 January for "making untrue comments" that had "severely disturbed the social order" and made to sign a statement of acknowledgment. It was reported on 7 February 2020 Li had died after contracting the disease from a patient in January 2020. His death triggered grief and anger on the social media, which became extended to demands for freedom of speech in China. China's anti-corruption body, the National Supervisory Commission, has initiated an investigation into the issues involving Li.

Local officials were criticised for hiding evidence of human-to-human transmission in early January, and suppressing reports about the disease during People's Congress meetings for political reasons. Criticism was directed at Hubei Governor Wang Xiaodong after he twice claimed at a press conference that 10.8 billion face masks were produced each year in the province, rather than the accurate number of 1.8 million.

Wuhan Police detained several Hong Kong media correspondents for over an hour when they were conducting interviews at Wuhan's Jinyintan Hospital on 14

January. Reports said the police brought the correspondents to a police station, where the police checked their travel documents and belongings, then asked them to delete video footage taken in the hospital before releasing them.

Authorities in Wuhan and Hubei provinces have been criticised for downplaying the severity of the outbreak and responding more slowly than they could have. The Beijing-based media journal, *Caixin* noted that Hubei did not roll out the first level of "public health emergency response mechanism" until 24 January, while several other provinces and cities outside the centre of the outbreak have already done so the day before. John Mackenzie, a senior expert at WHO, accused them of keeping "the figures quiet for a while because of some major meeting they had in Wuhan", alleging that there was a "period of very poor reporting, or very poor communication" in early January. On 19 January, four days before the city's lockdown, a *wan jia yan* was held in Wuhan, with over 40,000 families turning out; this attracted retrospective criticism.

The domestic *The Beijing News* argued that the local authorities should not have held such a public assembly while attempting to control the outbreak. The paper also stated that when their journalists visited the Huanan Seafood Wholesale Market where the coronavirus likely originated, most residents and merchants there were not wearing face masks. Zhou Xianwang, the mayor of Wuhan, later spoke to China Central Television, explaining that the banquet was held annually, that it is a "sample of the people's self-autonomy", and that the decision was made based on the fact that scientists then wrongly believed that the virus's ability to spread between humans was limited. Meanwhile, on 20 January, Wuhan's municipal department for culture and tourism gave out 200,000 tickets valid for visiting all tourist attractions in Wuhan to its citizens for free. The department was later criticised for disregarding the outbreak.

Tang Zhihong, the chief of the health department in Huanggang, was fired hours after she was unable to answer questions on how many people in her city were being treated.

Central government of China

In contrast to the widespread criticism of the local response, the central government has been praised by international experts and state media for its handling of the crisis. This has led to suggestions, in particular by the international media, that it is an attempt by the official press to shift public anger away from the central government and towards local authorities. It has been noted historically that the tendency of provincial governments to minimise reporting local incidents have been because of the central government directing a large proportion of the blame onto them. Critics, such as Wu Qiang, a former professor at Tsinghua University, and Steve Tsang, director of the China Institute at the University of London, have further argued the same point, with the latter suggesting that it was also exacerbated through local officials being "apprehensive about taking sensible preventive measures without knowing what Xi and other top leaders wanted as they feared that any missteps would have serious political consequences", a sentiment that Tsang argued was difficult to avoid when "power is concentrated in the hands of one top leader who is punitive to those who make mistakes".

Wuhan mayor Zhou Xianwang defended himself, referring to those suggestions by publicly blaming regulatory requirements that require local governments to first seek Beijing's approval, which delayed disclosure of the epidemic. He stated in an interview that "as a local government, we may disclose information only after we are given permission to do so. That is something that many people do not understand." The Chinese government has also been accused of rejecting help from the CDC and WHO.

Japanese government

The Japanese government has been criticized for its quarantine measures on the cruise Diamond Princess after the ship proved a fertile breeding ground for the virus. Kentaro Iwata, a infectious disease professor at Kobe University Hospital, said that the condition aboard was "completely chaotic" and "violating all infection control principles". On 22 February, the Ministry of Health, Labour and Welfare admitted that 23 passengers were disembarked without being properly tested for the virus. On 23 February, a Japanese female passenger tested positive after returning to her home in Tochigi Prefecture from the cruise ship. However, the woman was not among the 23 passengers.

South Korean government

On 22 February, the South Korean government apologized for calling the virus "Daegu Corona 19" in an offical report. The term has been widespread on social medias and rises concerns about discrimination.

Misinformation

After the initial outbreak, conspiracy theories and misinformation spread online regarding the origin and scale of the Wuhan coronavirus. Various social media posts claimed the virus was a bio-weapon, a population control scheme, or the result of a spy operation. Google, Facebook, and Twitter announced they will crack down on possible misinformation. In a blogpost, Facebook stated they would remove content flagged by leading global health organisations and local authorities that violate its content policy on misinformation leading to "physical harm".

On 2 February, the WHO declared there was a "massive infodemic" accompanying the outbreak and response, citing an over-abundance of reported information, accurate and false, about the virus that "makes it hard for people to find trustworthy sources and reliable guidance when they need it." The WHO stated that the high demand for timely and trustworthy information has incentivised the creation of a direct WHO 24/7 myth-busting hotline where its communication and social media teams have been monitoring and responding to misinformation through its website and social media pages. A group of scientists from outside China have released a statement to "strongly condemn" rumours and conspiracy theories about the origin of outbreak.

Xenophobia and racism

Since the outbreak of COVID-19, heightened prejudice, xenophobia and racism against peoples of Chinese and East Asian descent has arisen as a result, with incidents of fear, suspicion and hostility being noted across various countries. Although there has been support from Chinese both on and offline towards those in virus-stricken areas, many residents of Wuhan and Hubei have reported experiencing discrimination based on their regional origin.

On 30 January, WHO's Emergency Committee issued a statement advising all countries to be mindful of the "principles of Article 3 of the IHR," which cautions against "actions that promote stigma or discrimination," when conducting national response measures to the outbreak.

Open access of scientific papers

Owing to the urgency of the epidemic, many scientific publishers have made scientific papers related to the outbreak open access. Some scientists have chosen to share their results quickly on preprint servers such as BioRxiv, while archivists have created an illegal open access database of over 5,000 papers.

SOCIO-ECONOMIC IMPACT

The epidemic coincided with the Chunyun, a major travel season associated with the Chinese New Year holiday. A number of events involving large crowds were cancelled by national and regional governments, including annual New Year festivals, with private companies also independently closing their shops and tourist attractions such as Hong Kong Disneyland and Shanghai Disneyland. Many Lunar New Year events and tourist attractions have been closed to prevent mass gatherings, including the Forbidden City in Beijing and traditional temple fairs.

In 24 of China's 31 provinces, municipalities and regions, authorities extended the New Year's holiday to 10 February, instructing most workplaces not to re-open until that date. These regions represented 80% of the country's GDP and 90% of exports. Hong Kong raised its infectious disease response level to the highest and declared an emergency, closing schools until March and cancelling its New Year celebrations.

As Mainland China is a major economy and a manufacturing hub, the viral outbreak has been seen to pose a major destabilising threat to the global economy. Agathe Demarais of the Economist Intelligence Unit has forecast that markets will remain volatile until a clearer image emerges on potential outcomes. Some analysts have estimated that the economic fallout of the epidemic on global growth could surpass that of the SARS outbreak. Dr. Panos Kouvelis, director of "The Boeing Center" at Washington University in St. Louis, estimates a $300+ billion impact on world's supply chain that could last up to two years. Organization of the Petroleum Exporting Countries reportedly "scrambled" after a steep decline in oil prices due to lower demand from China.

The demand for personal protection equipment has risen 100-fold, according to WHO director-general Tedros Adhanom. This demand has lead to the increase in prices of up to twenty times the normal price and also induced delays on the supply of medical items for four to six months.

Mainland China

Tourism in China has been hit hard by travel restrictions and fears of contagion, including a ban on both domestic and international tour groups. Many airlines have either cancelled or greatly reduced flights to China and several travel advisories now warn against travel to China. Many countries, including France, Japan, Australia, New Zealand, the United Kingdom and the United States, have evacuated their nationals from the Wuhan and Hubei provinces.

The majority of schools and universities have extended their annual holidays to mid-February. Overseas students enrolled at Chinese universities have been returning home over fears of being infected—the first cases to be reported by Nepal and Kerala, a southern state of India, were both of students who had returned home.

The Finance Ministry of China announced it would fully subsidise personal medical cost incurred by patients.

CNN reported that some people from Wuhan "have become outcasts in their own country, shunned by hotels, neighbors and – in some areas – placed under controversial quarantine measures." Ian Lipkin, a Columbia University-based epidemiologist advising the Chinese authorities on handling the outbreak, opined that the barricades and signs forbidding entry to people from Wuhan as well as neighbourhood tips leading to involuntary quarantine were "probably" necessary due to the lack of other viable options.

The sale of new cars in China has been impacted due to the outbreak. There was a 92% reduction on the volume of cars sold during the first two weeks of February 2020.

Australia

Australia is expected to be one of three economies worst affected by the epidemic, along with Mainland China, and Hong Kong. Early estimations have GDP contracting by 0.2% to 0.5% and more than 20,000 Australian jobs being lost. The Australian Treasurer said that the country would no longer be able to promise a budget surplus due to the outbreak. The Australian dollar dropped to its lowest value since the Great Recession.

The Australasian College for Emergency Medicine called for a calm and a fact-based response to the epidemic, asking people to avoid racism, "panic and division" and the spread of misinformation. A large amount of protective face masks were purchased by foreign and domestic buyers, which has sparked a nationwide face masks shortage. In response to price increases of nearly 2000%, the Pharmaceutical Society of Australia has called on these "unethical suppliers" to keep supplies affordable.

Tourism bodies have suggested that the total economic cost to the sector, as of 11 February 2020, would be A$4.5bn. Casino earnings are expected to fall. At least two localities in Australia, Cairns and the Gold Coast, have reported already lost earnings of more that $600 million. The Australian Tourism Industry Council (ATIC) called on the Government of Australia for financial support especially in light of the large number of small businesses affected.

Mining companies are thought to be highly exposed to the outbreak, since sales to China constitute 93% of the sales of Fortescue Metals, 55% of the sales of BHP, and 45% of the sales of Rio Tinto. The iron ore shipping gauge dropped 99.9% as a result of the outbreak, and the virus has made shipping and logistic operations of mining companies more complicated.

Agriculture is also experiencing negative effects from the outbreak, including the Australian dairy industry, fishing industry, wine producers, and meat producers. On 13 February 2020 Rabobank, which specialises in agricultural banking, warned that the agricultural sector had eight weeks for the coronavirus to be contained before facing major losses.

The education sector is expected to suffer a US$5 billion loss according to an early government estimate, including costs due to "tuition fee refunds, free deferral of study, realignment of teaching calendars and student accommodation costs." The taxpayer is likely to be required to cover the shortfall in education budgets. An estimated 100,000 students were not able to enroll at the start of the semester. Nearly two-thirds of Chinese students were forced to remain overseas due to visa restrictions on travellers from Mainland China. Salvatore Babones, associate professor at the University of Sydney, stated that "Australia will remain an attractive study destination for Chinese students, but it may take several years for Chinese student numbers to recover".

Brazil

Two Brazilian banks predicted the deceleration of economic growth in China. UBS has reviewed its estimations from 6% to 5.4%, while Itaú stated a reduction to 5.8%. A representative of some of the bigger Brazilian companies of the electronics sector, Eletros, stated that the current stock for the supply of components is enough for around 10 to 15 days.

The prices of soy-beans, oil and iron ore have been falling. These three goods represent 30%, 24%, and 21% of the Brazilian exports to China, respectively.

Europe

At least ten towns in the Lombardy region of Italy were locked down following an outbreak, with at least 132 confirmed cases by 23 February. In the United Kingdom, digger manufacturer JCB announced that it plans to reduce working hours and production due to shortages in their supply chain caused by the outbreak.

In Spain, a large number of exhibitors (including Chinese firms Huawei and Vivo) announced plans to pull out of or reduce their presence at Mobile World Congress, a wireless industry trade show in Barcelona, Spain, due to concerns over coronavirus. On 12 February 2020, GSMA CEO John Hoffman announced that the event had been cancelled, as the concerns had made it "impossible" to host.

In Germany, according to the Deutsche Bank the outbreak of the novel coronavirus may contribute to a recession in Germany.

Owing to an increase in the demand for masks, on 1 February most masks were sold out in Portuguese pharmacies. On 4 February, President Marcelo Rebelo de Sousa admitted that the epidemic of the new coronavirus in China "affects the economic activity of a very powerful economy and thus affects the world's economic activity or could affect". He also admitted the possibility of economic upheavals due to the break in production."

Japan

Prime Minister Shinzô Abe has said that "the new coronavirus is having a major impact on tourism, the economy and our society as a whole". Face masks have sold out across the nation and stocks of face masks are depleted within a day of new arrivals. There has been pressure placed on the healthcare system as demands for medical checkups increase. Chinese people have reported increasing discrimination. The health minister has pointed out that the situation has not reached a point where mass gatherings must be called off.

Aviation, retail and tourism sectors have reported decreased sales and some manufactures have complained about disruption to Chinese factories, logistics and supply chains. Prime Minister Abe has considered using emergency funds to mitigate the outbreak's impact on tourism, of which Chinese nationals account for 40%. S&P Global noted that the worst hit shares were from companies spanning travel, cosmetics and retail sectors which are most exposed to Chinese tourism. Nintendo announced that they would delay shipment of the Nintendo Switch, which is manufactured in China, to Japan.

The outbreak itself has been a concern for the 2020 Summer Olympics which is scheduled to take place in Tokyo starting at the end of July. The national government has thus been taking extra precautions to help minimise the outbreak's impact. The Tokyo organising committee and the International Olympic Committee have been monitoring the outbreak's impact in Japan.

Hong Kong

Hong Kong has seen high-profile protests that saw tourist arrivals from Mainland China plummet over an eight-month period. The viral epidemic put additional pressure on the travel sector to withstand a prolonged period of downturn. A drop in arrivals from third countries more resilient during the previous months has also been cited as a concern. The city is already in recession and Moody has lowered the city's credit rating. The worst economic effects from the outbreak are expected for Australia, Hong Kong and China.

There has also been a renewed increase in protest activity as hostile sentiment against Mainland Chinese strengthened over fears of viral transmission from Mainland China, with many calling for the border ports to be closed and for all Mainland Chinese travellers to be refused entry.

Incidents have included a number of petrol bombs being thrown at police stations, a homemade bomb exploding in a toilet, and foreign objects being thrown onto transit rail tracks between Hong Kong and the Mainland Chinese border. Political issues raised have included concerns that Mainland Chinese may prefer to travel to Hong Kong to seek free medical help (which has since been addressed by the Hong Kong government).

Since the outbreak of the virus, a significant number of products have been sold out across the city, including face masks and disinfectant products (such as alcohol and bleach). An ongoing period of panic buying has also caused many stores to be cleared of non-medical products such as bottled water, vegetables and rice. The Government of Hong Kong had its imports of face masks cancelled as global face mask stockpiles decline.

In view of the coronavirus outbreak, the Education Bureau closed all kindergartens, primary schools, secondary schools and special schools until 17 February. This was later extended to 1 March due to further development of the epidemic. The disruption has raised concerns over the situation of students who are due to take examinations at the end of the year, especially in light of the protest-related disruption that happened in 2019.

On 5 February, flag carrier Cathay Pacific requested its 27,000 employees to voluntarily take three weeks of unpaid leave by the end of June. The airline had previously reduced flights to mainland China by 90% and to overall flights by 30%.

Macau

On 4 February 2020, all casinos in Macau were ordered to shut down for 15 days. All casinos reopened on 20 February 2020.

Southeast Asia

Among Association of Southeast Asian Nations countries, the city-state of Singapore was forecast to be one of the worst hit countries by Maybank. The tourism sector was considered to be an "immediate concern" along with the effects on production lines due to disruption to factories and logistics in mainland China. Singapore has witnessed panic buying of essential groceries, and of masks, thermometers and sanitation products despite being advised against doing so by the government. Prime Minister Lee Hsien Loong said that a recession in the country is a possibility, and that the country's economy "would definitely take a hit".

Maybank economists rated Thailand as being most at risk, with the threat of the viral outbreak's impact on tourism causing the Thai baht to fall to a seven-month low.

In Malaysia, economists predicted that the outbreak would affect the country's GDP, trade and investment flows, commodity prices and tourist arrivals. Initially, the cycling race event Le Tour de Langkawi was rumoured to be cancelled, but the organiser stated that it would continue to be held as usual. Despite this, two cycling teams, the Hengxiang Cycling Team and the Giant Cycling Team, both from

China, were pulled from participating in this race due to fear of the coronavirus outbreak. As the outbreak situation has worsened, some of the upcoming concerts held in Kuala Lumpur, such as Kenny G, Jay Chou, The Wynners, Super Junior, Rockaway Festival and Miriam Yeung, were postponed to a future date, and the upcoming Seventeen concert was cancelled.

In Indonesia, over 10,000 Chinese tourists cancelled trips and flights to major destinations such as Bali, Jakarta, Bandung, etc., over coronavirus fears. Many existing Chinese visitors are queuing up with the Indonesian authority appealing for extended stay.

Prime Minister Hun Sen of Cambodia made a special visit to China with an aim to showcase Cambodia's support to China in fighting the outbreak of the epidemic.

South Asia

In India, economists expect the near-term impact of the outbreak to be limited to the supply chains of major conglomerates, especially pharmaceuticals, fertilisers, automobiles, textiles and electronics. A severe impact on global trade logistics is also expected due to disruption of logistics in Mainland China, but due to the combined risk with regional geopolitical tensions, wider trade wars and Brexit.

In Sri Lanka, research houses expect the economic impact to be limited to a short term impact on the tourism and transport sectors.

South Korea

South Korea has been reporting increasing human-to-human community transmission of SARS-CoV-2 since 19 February 2020, traced to a church of Shincheonji, located near the city of Daegu. Apart from the city of Daegu and the church community involved, most of South Korea is operating close to normality, although nine planned festivals have been closed and tax-free retailers are closing. South Korean military manpower agency made an announcement that conscription from the Daegu will temporarily be suspended. The *Daegu Office of Education* decided to postpone the start of every school in the region by one week.

Numerous educational institutes have temporarily shut down, including dozens of kindergartens in Daegu and several elementary schools in Seoul. As of February 18, most universities in South Korea had announced plans to postpone the start of the spring semester. This included 155 universities planning to delay the semester start by 2 weeks to March 16, and 22 universities planning to delay the semester start by 1 week to March 9. Also, on 23 February 2020, all kindergartens, elementary schools, middle schools, and high schools were announced to delay the semester start from March 2 to March 9.

The economy of South Korea is forecast to grow 1.9%, which is down from 2.1%. The government has provided 136.7 billion won for local governments as support. The government has also organized the procurement of masks and other hygiene equipment.

Taiwan

On 24 January, the Taiwanese government announced a temporary ban on the export of face masks for a month, in order to secure a supply of masks for its own citizens. On 2 February 2020, Taiwan's Central Epidemic Command Center postponed the opening of primary and secondary schools until 25 February. Taiwan has also announced a ban of cruise ships from entering all Taiwanese ports. In January, Italy has banned flights from Mainland China, Hong Kong, Macau, and Taiwan. On 10 February, the Philippines announced it will ban the entry of Taiwanese citizens due to the One-China Policy. Later on 14 February, Presidential Spokesperson of Philippines, Salvador Panelo, announced the lifting of the temporary ban on Taiwan. In early February 2020 Taiwan's Central Epidemic Command Center requested the mobilisation of the Taiwanese Armed Forces in order to contain the spread of the virus and to build up the defences against it. Soldiers were dispatched to the factory floors of major mask manufacturers in order to help staff the 62 additional mask production lines being set up at the time.

In the aviation industry, Taiwanese carrier China Airlines's direct flights to Rome have been rejected and cancelled since Italy has announced the ban on Taiwanese flights. On the other hand, the second-largest Taiwanese carrier, Eva Air, has also postponed the launch of Milan and Phuket flights. Both Taiwanese airlines have cut numerous cross-strait destinations, leaving just three Chinese cities still served.

United States

The viral outbreak was cited by many companies in their briefings to shareholders, but several maintained confidence that they would not be too adversely affected by short-term disruption due to "limited" exposure to the Chinese consumer market. Those with manufacturing lines in mainland China warned about possible exposure to supply shortages.

Silicon Valley representatives expressed worries about serious disruption to production lines, as much of the technology sector relies on factories in Mainland China. Since there had been a scheduled holiday over Lunar New Year, the full effects of the outbreak on the tech sector were considered to be unknown as of 31 January 2020, according to *The Wall Street Journal.*

Cities with high populations of Chinese residents have seen an increase in demand for face masks to protect against the virus; many are purchasing masks to mail to relatives in Mainland China, Hong Kong, and Macau, where there is a shortage of masks. As of February 2020, many stores in the United States had sold out of masks. This mask shortage has caused an increase in prices.

Universities in the United States have warned about a significant impact to their income due to the large number of Chinese international students potentially unable to attend classes.

HOW THE CORONAVIRUS EPIDEMIC COULD UPEND THE GLOBAL ECONOMY

There are many ways to measure the costs of coronavirus. There have now been more than 24,000 officially reported cases, and nearly 500 people have died, but we'd be wise not to have much faith in these figures. A report from the Lancet estimated that as of Jan. 25 the true number of coronavirus cases in Hubei province, which includes the city of Wuhan, was not 761, as officially reported, but 75,815.

The impact on China's economy will be considerable. Quarantine and internal border controls have been imposed, and local officials are now overcompensating in response to criticism from Beijing that they were slow to respond to the initial outbreak. Businesses and schools are likely to remain closed for weeks. Economic activity in many Chinese cities is sharply reduced.

There is also the mounting economic cost for the entire global economy. The outbreak of severe acute respiratory syndrome (SARS) in 2003 knocked one to two percentage points off China's GDP that year, which then cost one-quarter to one-third of a percentage point in global growth, according to estimates. The larger number of infections from the coronavirus suggests the impact could be more severe this time for both China and the world. What happens in China matters more than ever for the rest of us. Its share of the global economy has surged from 8% in 2002 to 19% today, and it's now the world's second largest economy.

Companies in other countries dependent on Chinese supply chains are already facing a slowdown: Japan, Australia, New Zealand, Singapore, Italy and the U.S. have all imposed travel restrictions. Asian countries will see a sharp reduction in the number of arriving Chinese tourists, an important source of growth.

Oil prices have fallen 20% over the past month on expectations of lower demand from China and reduced sales of jet fuel as flights are grounded. Press reports suggest that China's daily crude-oil consumption has fallen by 20%, an amount equal to consumption in Britain and Italy combined. OPEC and Russian officials are now debating whether to cut oil production to buoy prices. Prices for metals and other construction materials have fallen.

This is also a hit to the "Phase 1" trade deal the U.S. and China concluded last month. China was already unlikely to purchase the additional $200 billion of U.S. goods over two years that it committed to buying. The slowdown will make that figure hard to achieve.

But the greatest cost will come to China's reputation as a reliable trade partner. In developed countries, health care systems are quick to identify public-health risks and better able to respond to them. China's top-down authoritarian political system makes things worse. In the early stages of these kinds of crises, local officials try to avoid blame from Beijing by hiding information about outbreaks and the extent to which health facilities are overmatched. In later stages of the crisis, they overcorrect to show Beijing they've taken charge of the problem.

In the process, China creates the impression that it has learned little since the SARS crisis, giving the rest of the world reason to try to reduce its dependence on China for growth and production.

We're moving closer to the day when it is China's increasingly hefty economy, not America's, that's most to blame for a global recession.

2

Coronavirus

Coronaviruses (CoV) are a large family of viruses that cause illness ranging from the common cold to more severe diseases such as Middle East Respiratory Syndrome (MERS-CoV) and Severe Acute Respiratory Syndrome (SARS-CoV). A novel coronavirus (nCoV) is a new strain that has not been previously identified in humans. Coronaviruses are zoonotic, meaning they are transmitted between animals and people. Detailed investigations found that SARS-CoV was transmitted from civet cats to humans and MERS-CoV from dromedary camels to humans. Several known coronaviruses are circulating in animals that have not yet infected humans.

Common signs of infection include respiratory symptoms, fever, cough, shortness of breath and breathing difficulties. In more severe cases, infection can cause pneumonia, severe acute respiratory syndrome, kidney failure and even death.

Standard recommendations to prevent infection spread include regular hand washing, covering mouth and nose when coughing and sneezing, thoroughly cooking meat and eggs. Avoid close contact with anyone showing symptoms of respiratory illness such as coughing and sneezing.

CORONAVIRUS DISEASE 2019

Coronavirus disease 2019 (COVID-19) is an infectious disease caused by SARS-CoV-2, a virus closely related to the SARS virus. The disease is the cause of the 2019–20 coronavirus outbreak. It is primarily spread between people via respiratory droplets from infected individuals when they cough or sneeze. Time from exposure to onset of symptoms is generally between 2 and 14 days. Spread can be limited by handwashing and other hygiene measures.

People may have few symptoms or develop fever, cough, and shortness of breath. Cases can progress to pneumonia and multi-organ failure. There is no vaccine or specific antiviral treatment, with management involving treatment of symptoms, supportive care, and experimental measures. The case fatality rate is estimated at between 1% to 3%.

Cases were initially identified in Wuhan, capital of Hubei province in China in December 2019. Cases reported outside China have predominantly been in people who have recently travelled to Mainland China, however a few cases of local transmission have also occurred. More than 2,300 deaths have been reported in Mainland China, and 15 deaths in other parts of the world.

The World Health Organization (WHO) and U.S. Centers for Disease Control (CDC) recommend that persons who suspect that they are carrying the virus wear a surgical face mask and seek medical advice by calling a doctor rather than directly visiting a clinic in person. Masks are not recommended for the general public. The WHO has declared the 2019–20 coronavirus outbreak to be a Public Health Emergency of International Concern (PHEIC). As of 19 February 2020, only Mainland China was listed as an area with known ongoing community spread of the disease.

Signs and symptoms

Those infected may either be asymptomatic or develop symptoms, including fever, cough or shortness of breath. Diarrhea or upper respiratory symptoms (e.g. sneezing, runny nose, sore throat) are less frequent. Cases can progress to pneumonia, multi-organ failure, and death. The length of the incubation period is estimated to be between two and ten days by the World Health Organization and between two and 14 days by the United States Centers for Disease Control and Prevention (CDC). A study had found rare cases where the incubation period was as long as 24 days.

Cause

The disease is caused by the virus severe acute respiratory syndrome coronavirus 2 (SARS-CoV-2), previously referred to as the 2019 novel coronavirus (2019-nCoV). The virus is thought to have an animal origin.

It is primarily spread between people via respiratory droplets from the coughs and sneezes. Officials in Shanghai confirmed several transmission modes, including direct transmission, contact transmission and aerosol transmission, the latter two involving transmission when someone touches a surface contaminated with tainted respiratory droplets and inhalation of air contaminated with tainted respiratory droplets.

An epidemiological study of the first 72,314 cases suggested that there may have been a "continuous common source" of the outbreak in December 2019, which would imply that several animal to human zoonotic events occurred at the Huanan Seafood Wholesale Market. According to this theory, the primary source of infection became human-to-human transmission in early January 2020.

Diagnosis

The WHO has published several testing protocols for the disease. Testing uses real time reverse transcription-polymerase chain reaction (rRT-PCR). The test can be done on respiratory or blood samples. Results are generally available within a few hours to days. Chinese scientists were able to isolate a strain of the coronavirus and publish the genetic sequence so that laboratories across the world could independently develop PCR tests to detect infection by the virus. Diagnostic guidelines released by Zhongnan Hospital of Wuhan University suggested methods for detecting infections based upon clinical features and epidemiological risk. These involved identifying patients who had at least two of the following symptoms in addition to a history of travel to Wuhan or contact with other infected patients: fever, imaging features of pneumonia, normal or reduced white blood cell count, or reduced lymphocyte count.

Prevention

Global health organisations have published preventive measures to reduce the chances of infection. Recommendations are similar to those published for other coronaviruses: frequent washing of hands with soap and water; not touching the eyes, nose, or mouth with unwashed hands; and practicing good respiratory hygiene.

The use of masks by healthy members of the public is not recommended outside of China.

To prevent transmission, the CDC recommends that infected individuals stay at home except to get medical care; call ahead before visiting a healthcare provider; wear a facemask (especially in public); cover coughs and sneezes with a tissue; regularly wash hands with soap and water; and avoid sharing personal household items.

No vaccine currently exists against SARS-CoV-2.

Management

There are no specific antiviral medications approved for this disease. Symptoms are managed with supportive care. The WHO has published detailed treatment recommendations for hospitalized patients with severe acute respiratory infection (SARI) when a SARS-CoV-2 infection is suspected. The WHO also recommended volunteers take part in randomized controlled trials for testing the effectiveness and safety of potential treatments.

The Beijing branch of China's National Health Commission suggested the use of lopinavir/ritonavir as part of treatment plans in the absence of an approved drug for this indication. The lopinavir/ritonavir combination and interferon can now be claimed for via health insurance in some countries.

Psychological

Infected individuals may experience distress from quarantine, travel restrictions, side effects of treatment, or fear of the infection itself. To address these concerns, the National Health Commission of China published a national guideline for psychological crisis intervention on 27 January 2020.

Alternative medicine

Chinese health authorities recommend the use of traditional Chinese medicine (TCM) in addition to standard medical supportive care to prevent or treat the disease. On 22 January, National Health Commission put TCM into the third issue of the COVID diagnostic and treatment plan. On 2 February, Wuhan officials ordered all patients to be put on a specific TCM treatment. On 14 February, Wuhan opened a TCM-oriented temporary hospital. The efficacy and safety of TCM has not been established in coronavirus infections.

Prognosis

According to WHO, based on analysis of 44,000 cases of COVID-19 in Hubei province, around 80% of patients only have a mild form of the disease, 14% developed more severe disease such as pneumonia, 5% have critical disease, and 2% of cases are fatal. Among those who died initially, many had preexisting conditions, including hypertension, diabetes, or cardiovascular disease, and the median time from initial symptoms to death was 14 days (range 6-41 days).

Epidemiology

Overall mortality and morbidity rates due to infection are not well established; while the case fatality rate changes over time in the current outbreak, the proportion of infections that progress to diagnosable disease remains unclear. However, preliminary research has yielded case fatality rate numbers between 2% and 3%; in January 2020 the WHO suggested that the case fatality rate was approximately 3%, and 2% in February 2020 in Hubei.

An unreviewed preprint study by Imperial College London among 55 fatal cases noted that early estimates of mortality may be too high as asymptomatic infections are missed. They estimated a mean infection fatality ratio (the mortality among infected) ranging from 0.8% when including asymptomatic carriers to 18% when including only symptomatic cases from Hubei province.

Research

Vaccine

Many organizations are using published genomes to develop possible vaccines against SARS-CoV-2. Bodies developing vaccines include the Chinese Center for Disease Control and Prevention, the University of Hong Kong, and Shanghai East Hospital. Three vaccine projects are being supported by the Coalition for Epidemic Preparedness Innovations (CEPI), including projects by the biotechnology companies Moderna and Inovio Pharmaceuticals and another by the University of Queensland. The United States National Institutes of Health (NIH) is cooperating with Moderna to create an RNA vaccine matching a spike of the coronavirus surface, and intends to start human trials by May 2020. Inovio Pharmaceuticals is developing a DNA-based vaccination and collaborating with a Chinese firm, hoping to perform human trials in the summer of 2020. In Australia, the University of Queensland is investigating the potential of a molecular clamp vaccine that would genetically modify viral proteins in order to stimulate an immune reaction. In Canada, the International Vaccine Centre (VIDO-InterVac), University of Saskatchewan, are working on a vaccine, aiming to start animal testing in March 2020 and human testing in 2021.

In January 2020, Janssen Pharmaceutical Companies began work on developing a vaccine, utilizing the same technologies used to make its experimental Ebola vaccine. In the following month, the U.S. Department of Health and Human Services' Biomedical Advanced Research and Development Authority (BARDA) announced that it would collaborate with Janssen and, later, Sanofi Pasteur (the vaccine division of Sanofi) to develop a vaccine. Sanofi has previously worked on a vaccine for SARS and it stated to expect to have a vaccine candidate within six months that could be ready to test in people within a year to 18 months.

Antiviral

No drug has yet been approved to treat coronavirus infections in humans. Research into potential treatments for the disease was initiated in January 2020, and several antiviral drugs are already in clinical trials. Although completely new drugs may take until 2021 to develop, several of the drugs being tested are already approved for other antiviral indications, or are already in advanced testing.

Antivirals being tested include chloroquine; darunavir; galidesivir; interferon beta; the lopinavir/ritonavir combination; the RNA polymerase inhibitor remdesivir; and triazavirin. Arbidol and Darunavir were proposed by the National Health Commission. Preliminary results from a multicentric trial, announced in a press conference and described by Jianjun, Zhenxue and Xu, suggested that chloroquine is effective and safe in treating COVID-19 associated pneumonia, "improving lung imaging findings, promoting a virus-negative conversion, and shortening the disease course". The authors stated that chloroquine is recommended for inclusion in the *Guidelines for the Prevention, Diagnosis, and Treatment of Pneumonia Caused by COVID-19* issued by the Chinese National Health Commission for treatment of COVID-19 infection in larger populations. Jianjun, Zhenxue and Xu listed 15 trials formally registered with the Chinese Clinical Trial Registry, including a randomised trial in Wuhan of two groups of 100 patients on different dosages versus a group of 100 on a placebo, and a randomised trial in Shanghai of 100 patients taking oral hydroxychloroquine sulfate tablets versus 100 taking placebos.

Terminology

The World Health Organization on 11 February 2020 announced that "COVID-19" will be the official name of the disease. World Health Organization chief Tedros Adhanom Ghebreyesus said "co" stands for "corona", "vi" for "virus" and "d" for "disease", while "19" was for the year, as the outbreak was first identified on December 31. Tedros said the name had been chosen to avoid references to a specific geographical location (i.e. China), animal species or group of people in line with international recommendations for naming aimed at preventing stigmatization.

TIMELINE OF THE 2019–20 CORONAVIRUS OUTBREAK IN DECEMBER 2019 – JANUARY 2020

The chronology and epidemiology of SARS-CoV-2, the virus responsible for the 2019–20 coronavirus outbreak originating in Wuhan, China. It may not include all contemporary major responses and measures. Furthermore, some developments may become known or fully understood only in retrospect. (This omnibus timeline is divided into monthly sections and articles: This chronological section covers December 2019 and January 2020, the next February 2020, and so on.)

Outbreak chronology

1–18 December 2019

On 31 December 2019, a consortium of Chinese medical experts were charged by the Chinese CDC with investigating the inception of what was commonly known as

Wuhan coronavirus. On 24 January 2020, their report was published in *The Lancet*. They noted from their review of local medical records that the first person later to be diagnosed with the Wuhan Coronavirus had first presented with symptoms on 8 December 2019. However, the consortium found an earlier case of a person who had first experienced symptoms on 1 December 2019, pointing to an even earlier origin. Apart from this early case, between 8 and 18 December 2019, seven cases later diagnosed with Wuhan coronavirus were documented, two of them were linked with the Huanan Seafood Wholesale Market of Wuhan, five were not.

12 December 2019

Chinese state broadcaster CCTV reported in a broadcast airing on 12 January 2020 that a "new viral outbreak was first detected in the city of Wuhan, China, on 12 December 2019."

21 December 2019

Chinese epidemiologists with the Chinese Center for Disease Control (CDC) published an article on 1 January 2020 stating that the first cluster of patients with "pneumonia of an unknown cause" had been identified on 21 December 2019.

24 December 2019

Singapore's Ministry of Health (MOH) reported that the first case of what would later be named the 2019-nCov (Wuhan Coronavirus) had been diagnosed. It was later confirmed to not actually be related to the outbreak.

29 December 2019

According to a CDC publication on 31 January 2020, the facts leading up to the identification of the 2019-nCoV were as follows, "On 29 December 2019, a hospital in Wuhan admitted four individuals with pneumonia and recognized that all four had worked in the Huanan Seafood Wholesale Market, which sells live poultry, aquatic products, and several kinds of wild animals to the public.

The hospital reported this occurrence to the local center for disease control (CDC), which lead Wuhan CDC staff to initiate a field investigation with a retrospective search for pneumonia patients potentially linked to the market. The investigators found additional patients linked to the market, and on 30 December, health authorities from Hubei Province reported this cluster to China CDC. The following day, China CDC sent experts to Wuhan to support the investigation and control effort. Samples from these patients were obtained for laboratory analyses."

30 December 2019

On 30 December 2019, Dr. Li Wenliang, an ophthalmologist at Wuhan Central Hospital in Wuhan, China, posted a warning to alumni from his medical school class via a WeChat online forum that a cluster of seven patients treating within the ophthalmology department had been unsuccessfully treated for symptoms of viral pneumonia and diagnosed with SARS. Because these patients did not respond to traditional treatments, they were quarantined in an ER department of the Wuhan Central Hospital. In the WeChat forum, Li posted that this cluster of patients appeared to be infected by SARS. Dr. Li posted a snippet of an RNA analysis finding "SARS coronavirus" and extensive bacteria colonies in a patient's airways according to a chat transcript that he and other chat members later shared online. (Dr. Li contracted this coronavirus from a patient he treated, was hospitalized on 12 January 2020 and died on 6 February 2020. Due to public outcry directed to the CCP outlets retracted original reports, while international news agents corrected reports published on the 6th stating the death on 7th. The official date of death was later announced as 7 February 2020. Dr. Li is widely known for the statement he gave before his death exemplifying how the Chinese government botched the containment of the Wuhan Coronavirus, stating "There should be more than one voice in a healthy society.")

The Chinese National Health Commission announced later that evening that 8 doctors engaging in this WeChat forum had been arrested by Wuhan Police and charged with "Ilegal acts of fabricating, spreading rumors and disrupting social order..."

Wuhan medical authorities forbade doctors from making public announcements and ordered them to report cases internally.

News of an outbreak of "pneumonia of unknown origin" started circulating on social media on the evening of 30 December 2019. The social media reports stated that 27 patients in Wuhan - most of them stall holders at the Huanan Seafood Market - had been treated for the mystery illness.

On the evening of 30 December 2019, an "urgent notice on the treatment of pneumonia of unknown cause" was issued by the Wuhan Municipal Health Committee on its Weibo social media account. It was reported that since the beginning of December, there had been "a successive series of patients with unexplained pneumonia" - 27 suspected cases in total, seven of which were in critical condition and 18 were stable, two of which were on the verge of being discharged soon. The Wuhan Municipal Health Committee reported to the WHO that 27 people had been diagnosed with pneumonia of unknown cause. Most were stallholders from the Huanan Seafood

Wholesale Market, seven of whom were in critical condition. The Wuhan Municipal Health Commission also made a public announcement regarding the situation.

Early investigations into the cause of the pneumonia ruled out seasonal flu, SARS, MERS and bird flu.

Hong Kong Secretary for Food and Health Sophia Chan Siu-chee announced after an urgent night-time meeting with officials and experts, "[any suspected cases] including the presentation of fever and acute respiratory illness or pneumonia, and travel history to Wuhan within 14 days before onset of symptoms, we will put the patients in isolation."

31 December 2019

On 31 December 2019, an "urgent notice on the treatment of pneumonia of unknown cause" was issued to the Wuhan Municipal Health Center.

As a result of the official announcement of the Wuhan Municipal Health Commission, Hong Kong, Macau and Taiwan immediately tightened their inbound screening processes.

Qu Shiqian, a vendor at the Huanan Seafood Market, said government officials had disinfected the premises on 31 December 2019 and told stallholders to wear masks. Qu said he had only learnt of the pneumonia outbreak from media reports. "Previously I thought they had flu," he said. "It should be not serious. We are fish traders. How can we get infected?"

"Chinese state television reported that a team of experts from the National Health Commission had arrived in Wuhan on 31 December 2019 to lead the investigation, while the People's Daily said the exact cause remained unclear and it would be premature to speculate." Chinese state broadcaster CCTV reported that a team of senior health experts had been dispatched to the city of Wuhan and were reported to be "conducting relevant inspection and verification work."

Tao Lina, a public health expert and former official with Shanghai's Centre for disease control and prevention, said, "I think we are [now] quite capable of killing it in the beginning phase, given China's disease control system, emergency handling capacity and clinical medicine support."

1 January

According to the Chinese state-sponsored Xinhua News, the Huanan Seafood Market was closed on 1 January 2020 for "regulation." However, in the Consortium's report of 24 January 2020, it was stated that the Huanan Seafood Market had been closed on 1 January 2020 for "cleaning and disinfection."

2 January

On 2 January, 41 admitted hospital patients in Wuhan, China, were confirmed to have contracted (laboratory-confirmed) the 2019-nCoV (Wuhan Coronavirus); 27 (66%) patients had direct exposure to Huanan Seafood Wholesale Market. All 41 patients were subsequently relocated from the hospital they had originally been diagnosed in to the Jin Yin-tan Hospital in Wuhan, China.

3 January

On 3 January 2020, Chinese scientists at the National Institute of Viral Disease Control and Prevention (IVDC) determined the genetic sequence of the novel â-genus coronaviruses (naming it '2019-nCoV') from specimens collected from patients in Wuhan, China, and three distinct strains were established.

Health authorities in Wuhan reported 44 cases, a big jump from the 27 reported on Tuesday. Eleven of the 44 were seriously ill, the Wuhan Municipal Health Commission said, although there had been no reported deaths to date. The health of the 121 close contacts of the cases was being monitored.

On 3 January 2020, Dr. Li Wenliang, the Wuhan ophthalmologist who had been arrested for spreading false "rumors" on WeChat, was summoned to the Wuhan Public Security Bureau where he was told to sign an official confession and admonition letter promising to cease spreading false "rumors" regarding the coronavirus. In the letter, he was accused of "making false comments" that had "severely disturbed the social order". The letter stated, "We solemnly warn you: If you keep being stubborn, with such impertinence, and continue this illegal activity, you will be brought to justice - is that understood?" Dr. Li signed the confession writing: "Yes, I understand." Li would later be supported e.g. in a blog run by China's Supreme People's Court on 28 January 2020. On 7 February 2020, Chinese state-sponsored news reported that Dr. Li had died from complications arising from his infection to the Wuhan coronavirus only to later delete the post and report Dr. Li as being in critical condition. He was subsequently confirmed the same day as having regrettably indeed deceased. Dr. Li is now being heralded as a whistleblower who exposed the Chinese government's early efforts to cover up the seriousness of the coronavirus pandemic which resulted in its rapid spread across China and the world.

4 January

The head of the University of Hong Kong's Centre for Infection, Ho Pak-leung, warned that the city should implement the strictest possible monitoring system for a mystery new viral pneumonia that infected dozens of people on the mainland, as it was highly possible that the illness was spreading from human to human. The microbiologist also warned that there could be a surge in cases during the upcoming Chinese New Year. Ho said he hoped the mainland would release more details as soon as possible about the patients infected with the disease, such as their medical history, to help experts analyse the illness and to allow for more effective preventive measures to be put in place.

The Singapore Ministry of Health said on Saturday, January 4, that it had been notified of the first suspected case of the "mystery Wuhan virus" in Singapore, involving a three-year-old girl from China who had pneumonia and a travel history to the Chinese city of Wuhan. On January 5, the Singapore Ministry of Health released a press statement stating that the earlier suspected case was not linked to the pneumonia cluster in Wuhan and was also tested negative for the SARS and MERS-CoV.

Chinese officials were criticized for failing do disclose any information about the "mysterious virus" that machine translations of official reports suggested may be caused by a new coronavirus.

The WHO waited for China to release information about the "mysterious new pneumonia virus". The United Nations agency activated its incident-management system at the country, regional and global level and was standing ready to launch a broader response if it was needed. The WHO's regional office in Manila said in Twitter posts Saturday.: "#China has reported to WHO regarding a cluster of pneumonia cases in Wuhan, Hubei Province. The Govt has also met with our country office,and updated @WHO on the situation. Govt actions to control the incident have been instituted and investigations into the cause are ongoing."

The Wuhan Institute of Virology didn't respond to an emailed request for comment on the infectious source.

5 January

The number of suspected cases reached 59 with seven in a critical condition. All were quarantined and local medical officials commenced the monitoring of 163 of their contacts. At this time, there had been no reported cases of human-to-human transmission or presentations in healthcare workers.

6 January

On Monday, January 6, the Wuhan health authorities announced they continued seeking the cause but had so far ruled out influenza, avian influenza, adenovirus, and coronaviruses SARS and MERS as the respiratory pathogen that had infected 59 people as of 5 January.

7 January

Since the outburst of social media discussion of the mysterious pneumonia outbreak in Wuhan, China, Chinese authorities censored the hashtag #WuhanSARS and were now investigating anyone who was allegedly spreading misleading information about the outbreak on social media.

The world continued to wait for China to disclose more information about what had triggered an unexplained pneumonia outbreak in Wuhan, China's tenth-largest city. "The U.S. Centers for Disease Control and Prevention (CDC) issued a travel notice Monday for travelers to Wuhan, Hubei province, China due to the cluster of cases of pneumonia of an unknown etiology..."

8 January

Scientists in China announced the discovery of a new coronavirus.

South Korea announced first possible case of virus coming from China. South Korea put a 36-year-old Chinese woman under isolated treatment amid concerns that she had brought back a form of viral pneumonia that had sickened dozens in mainland China and Hong Kong in the previous weeks. The unidentified woman, who worked for a South Korean company near capital Seoul, had experienced cough and fever since returning from a five-day trip to China on 30 December, the KCDC said in a press release. The woman had spent time in Wuhan, China, but had not visited the Huanan Seafood Market.

9 January

The WHO confirmed that the novel coronavirus had been isolated from one person who had been hospitalised. On the same day, the European Centre for Disease Prevention and Control posted its first risk assessment. The WHO also reported that Chinese authorities had acted swiftly, identifying the novel coronavirus within weeks of the onset of the outbreak, with the total number of positively tested people being 41. The first death from the virus occurred in a 61-year-old man who was a regular customer at the market. He had several significant medical conditions, including chronic liver disease, and died from heart failure and pneumonia. The incident was reported in China by the health commission via Chinese state media on 11 January.

Chinese scientists reported on Chinese state broadcaster CCTV that they had found a new "coronavirus in 15 of 57 patients with the illness in the central city of Wuhan, saying it has been preliminarily identified as the pathogen for the outbreak". The scientists announced that the current 'Wuhan Virus', a coronavirus, appears to not be as lethal as SARS. They reported that the new viral outbreak was first detected in the city of Wuhan on 12 December 2019. Additionally, a total of 59 people have been identified as contracting the illness, seven patients had been in a critical condition at some stage, and no healthcare workers were reported as having been infected.

11–12 January

In China, more than 700 close contacts of the 41 confirmed cases, including more than 400 healthcare workers, had been monitored, with no new cases reported in China since 5 January. The WHO published initial guidance on travel advice, testing in the laboratory and medical investigation.

13 January

The USCDC announced that the genome had been posted on the NIH genetic sequence database, GenBank. On the same day, Thailand witnessed the first confirmed case of 2019-nCoV, the first outside China. The affected 61-year-old Chinese woman, who is a resident of Wuhan, had not visited the Huanan Seafood Wholesale Market, but was noted to have been to other markets. She had arrived in Bangkok on 8 January.

14 January

On 14 January, two of the 41 confirmed cases in Wuhan were reported to include a married couple, raising the possibility of human-to-human transmission.

15 January

A second death occurred in a 69-year-old man in China on 15 January. The WHO published a protocol on diagnostic testing for 2019-nCoV, developed by a virology team from Charité Hospital.

16 January

On 16 January, the WHO was alerted by Japan's Ministry of Health, Labour and Welfare that a 30-year-old male Chinese national had tested positive to 2019-nCoV during a hospital stay between 10 and 15 January. He had not visited the Huanan Seafood Wholesale Market, but possibly had close contact with an affected person in Wuhan.

17 January

On 17 January, Thailand's second confirmed case was reported in a 74-year-old woman who arrived in Bangkok on a flight from Wuhan. The number of laboratory-confirmed cases rose to 45 in China.

Yang Xiaobo, head of the Assets Supervision and Administration Commission, died of pneumonia caused by the virus on 17 January.

18 January

After the first 41 laboratory-confirmed cases were identified on January 2, 2020, Chinese officials announced no new cases for the next 16 days, then reported 17 additional laboratory-confirmed cases, three of which were in critical condition. This brought the number of laboratory-confirmed cases in China to 62. The patients' ages ranged from 30 to 79. 19 were discharged and eight remain critical.

On the same day, the Wuhan City government held an annual banquet in the Baibuting community celebrating the Chinese New Year with forty thousand families in attendance despite the officials' knowledge of the spread of the Wuhan Coronavirus. They shared meals, plates and ate together. On 21 January 2020 when Wuhan mayor Zhou Xianwang was asked on state television why this banquet was held even after the number of cases had risen to 312 he responded, "The reason why the Baibuting community continued to host the banquet this year was based on the previous judgment that the spread of the epidemic was limited between humans, so there was not enough warning."

19 January

On 19 January, the first confirmed cases were reported in China, outside Wuhan, one in the southern province of Guangdong and two in Beijing. Wuhan reported 136 additional laboratory-confirmed cases, bringing the total number of laboratory-confirmed cases in China to 201. A new death was also reported in Wuhan, bringing the total number of fatalities in China to three.

20 January

Scientists from the China CDC identified three different strains of the 2019-nCoV confirming that the original Wuhan Coronavirus had mutated into two additional strains.

Chinese premier Li Keqiang urged decisive and effective efforts to prevent and control the epidemic. First confirmed case reported in South Korea. Beijing and Guangdong reported an additional three and thirteen laboratory-confirmed cases, respectively. Shanghai confirms its first case, bringing the total number of laboratory-confirmed cases in China to 218. The investigation team from China's National Health Commission confirmed for the first time that the coronavirus can be transmitted between humans. At least two people had become infected whilst living hundreds of miles from Wuhan.

Five attendees of an as-yet-unnamed private international sales company meeting of 109 attendees, 94 from overseas, held from January 20–22 at the Grand Hyatt Hotel, Singapore were diagnosed with the Wuhan Caronavirus upon returning home: one from Malaysia, two from South Korea and two from Singapore. One of the attendees was from Wuhan, China. It was reported that the company held a buffet for their delegates. These four diagnoses were not reported until February 5, 2020. The first laboratory-confirmed case in Singapore of an unrelated 67 year-old native of Wuhan was not reported until 23 January 2020. These cases linked to the meeting were the first evidence that the Wuhan Caronavirus had spread through human-to-human contact outside China, which the WHO has said is deeply concerning and could signal evidence of a much larger outbreak. As of February 5, 2020, the sister of a Malaysian who attended the meeting had been infected and four more local staff in Singapore were confirmed as having virus symptoms.

21 January

A total of 291 cases have now been reported across major cities in China, including Beijing and Shanghai. Howeverm most patients are in Wuhan, the central city of 11 million at the heart of the outbreak.

A report by the MRC Centre for Global Infectious Disease Analysis at Imperial College London suggested there could be more than 1,700 infections. However, Gabriel Leung, the dean of medicine at the University of Hong Kong, put the figure closer to 1,300.

After 300 confirmed diagnoses and 6 deaths, Chinese state media warned lower-level officials not to cover up the spread of a new coronavirus. Officials declared that anyone who concealed new cases would "be nailed on the pillar of shame for eternity", the political body responsible for law and order said. Local Chinese officials initially withheld information about the epidemic from the public. It later vastly under-reported the number of people that had been infected, downplayed the risks and failed to provide timely information that experts say could have saved lives. In its commentary published online on Tuesday January 20, 2020, the Communist Party's Central Political and Legal Commission talked of China having learned a "painful lesson" from the Sars epidemic and called for the public to be kept informed. Deception, it warned, could "turn a controllable natural disaster into a man-made disaster".

The Wuhan Municipal Health Commission reported at least 15 medical workers in Wuhan have also been infected with the virus, with one in a critical condition.

WHO Situation Report 1: (Please note that the WHO Situation Reports as official reportage stand on their own.)

Confirmed cases were reported in several new locations in China. Zhejiang province and Tianjin reported five and two laboratory-confirmed cases, respectively. Guangdong reported three additional laboratory-confirmed cases. Shanghai and Henan province reported an additional four and one laboratory-confirmed cases, respectively. One laboratory-confirmed case was reported in Sichuan province, and Chongqing reported five laboratory-confirmed cases. Shandong, Hunan, and Yunnan all reported one laboratory-confirmed case each. Jiangxi reported two laboratory-confirmed cases. The total number of laboratory-confirmed cases in China increased to 312 and the death toll increased to six.

New cases were also reported outside of mainland China. Taiwan reported its first laboratory-confirmed case, and the United States reported its first laboratory-confirmed case in the state of Washington, the first in North America.

China's Wuhan Institute filed to patent the use of Gilead's remdesivir for the treatment of novel coronavirus.

22 January

New cases: Macau and Hong Kong reported their first laboratory-confirmed cases, with Hong Kong reporting its second on the evening of 22 January. Beijing reported an additional five laboratory-confirmed cases, while Guangdong reported an additional nine laboratory-confirmed cases. Shanghai reported an additional five laboratory-confirmed cases, while Tianjin reported an additional two laboratory-confirmed cases. Zhejiang and Jiangxi reported an additional five and one laboratory-confirmed cases, respectively. Liaoning reported its first two laboratory-confirmed cases. Guizhou, Fujian, Anhui, Shanxi and Ningxia reported one laboratory-confirmed case each. Hainan reported four laboratory-confirmed cases. Hunan reported three additional laboratory-confirmed cases. Guangxi reported two laboratory-confirmed cases. In all, the total number of laboratory-confirmed cases in China increased to 571 and the death toll to 17.

Internationally, two more laboratory-confirmed cases were reported in Thailand, raising the total number of laboratory-confirmed cases in Thailand to four.

New data showed indications of the current rapid spread of the disease and an increase in the rate of transmission.

Officials announce a quarantine of the greater Wuhan, China area to commence 23 January 2020 at 10:00 am. No traffic will be allowed in or out of the city.

23 January

WHO Situation Report 3: Jiangsu reported its first laboratory-confirmed case.

Heilongjiang reported its first two laboratory-confirmed cases. Both Fujian and Guangxi reported an additional three laboratory-confirmed cases each. Shanghai reported an additional seven laboratory-confirmed cases. Xinjiang reported two laboratory-confirmed cases. Shaanxi reported three laboratory-confirmed cases. Gansu reported two laboratory-confirmed cases. Macau also reported its second laboratory-confirmed case, another 66-year-old man from Wuhan. In all, the total number of laboratory-confirmed cases in mainland China increased to 628 while the death toll remained at 17.

Singapore reported its first laboratory-confirmed case, a 66-year-old man from China. Vietnam confirmed its first two laboratory-confirmed cases, a 65 or 66-year-old father and 27 or 28-year-old son from China.

Wuhan suspended all public transportation from 10 a.m. onwards, including all bus, metro and ferry lines. Additionally, all outbound trains and flights were halted.

24 January

WHO Situation Report 4: 'Hong Kong confirms two new cases of pneumonia' - video news report from China News Service, January 24, 2020 (Captions available in English)

Shandong reported six additional laboratory-confirmed cases. Hunan reported 15 additional laboratory-confirmed cases. Liaoning reported one additional laboratory-confirmed case. Fujian reported four additional laboratory-confirmed cases. Anhui reported six additional laboratory-confirmed cases. Ningxia reported one additional laboratory-confirmed case. Shanghai reported 13 additional laboratory-confirmed cases, bringing the total up to 33.

Japan, South Korea, and the United States all confirmed their second cases. Singapore confirmed its second and third cases. Thailand confirmed its fifth case. Hong Kong confirmed three additional cases, bringing the total number to five. Nepal confirmed its first case, a student who returned from Wuhan. France reported its first three confirmed cases, the first occurrences in the EU. The French Health Minister Agnès Buzyn stated that it is likely other cases would arise in the country.

The first confirmed incidence of human-to-human transmission outside of China was documented by the WHO in Vietnam.

A study by Chinese researchers indicates that people can be symptom-free for several days while the coronavirus is incubating, increasing the risk of contagious infection without forewarning signs.

By the end of the day, the entire Hubei province have come under a city-by-city quarantine, apart from Xiangyang and Shennongjia Forestry District.

25 January

Chinese Communist Party general secretary Xi Jinping called the "accelerating spread" of the coronavirus a "grave situation" on the Party Politburo meeting, and that it was "mutating" as Beijing escalates measures to contain the illness.

WHO Situation Report 5: Australia confirmed its first four cases, one in Victoria and three in New South Wales. Malaysia reported its first three cases in Johor Bahru, and a fourth case later. Japan confirmed its third case. Canada confirmed its first case in Toronto. Thailand added two new cases for a total of seven. Singapore confirmed their fourth case.

A Chinese and a Sri Lankan suspected with the infection were admitted to a hospital in Sri Lanka.

Liang Wudong, a 62-year-old doctor, reportedly died in the Hubei province from the coronavirus.

26 January

WHO Situation Report 6: The Spring Festival holiday was extended to contain coronavirus outbreak.

Shanghai reported its first death, an 88-year-old man.

The United States confirmed its third, fourth, and fifth cases: two in California and one in Arizona. Macau confirmed three additional cases, bringing its total to five. Hong Kong confirmed its sixth, seventh, and eighth cases. Thailand has confirmed its eighth case. The first of five patients was already discharged. There are another 39 suspected cases awaiting confirmation.

The Chinese Center for Disease Control and Prevention (CCDC) has started developing vaccines against the coronavirus, an official with the center said on Sunday.

Health officials in Ivory Coast are dealing with a suspected case of coronavirus, the country's health ministry has announced.

The United Nation's WHO Director-General Tedros Ghebreyesus said he was on his way to Beijing to confer with Chinese officials and health experts about the coronavirus outbreak.

China started requiring nationwide use of monitoring stations for screening, identification and immediate isolation of coronavirus-infected travellers, including at airports, railway stations, bus stations and ports.

A tentative clinical profile for the new coronavirus (2019-nCoV) was published by an assistant professor of population health science at the Icahn School of

Medicine at Mount Sinai in New York. The lethality of the virus is unknown; however, the death toll has now climbed to above three percent.

Wang Xianliang, a Hubei provincial government official, died of pneumonia caused by the virus.

27 January

WHO Situation Report 7: Dr. Gabriel Leung, Dean of the University of Hong Kong medical school and one of the foremost world experts on SARS and viruses, gave a three-hour presentation published on YouTube wherein he made nowcasts and forecasts of the Wuhan Virus Pandemic. Using traditional scientific modeling techniques that predict the spread of viruses, Dr. Leung projected the true number of coronavirus infections was likely 10 time more than the official reported numbers. Dr. Leung estimated that there were between 44,000-100,000 infections in China as of 24 January 2020. He stated that draconian measures were needed to slow the progress of the virus but that these measures would have no effect in stopping the coronavirus pandemic. He projected that the number of infections would continue exponentially peaking out in late April or May 2020. Dr. Leung predicted that at the peak of the pandemic, there could be up to 100,000 new infections per day. Dr. Leung subsequently published an article in The Lancet nowcasting and forecasting the likely progression of the Wuhan Coronavirus taking into consideration numerous variables. Zhou Xianwang, the mayor of Wuhan, said on a Chinese state television talkshow that rules imposed by Beijing limited what he could disclose about the threat posed by the Wuhan Coronavirus as it unfolded, suggesting "the central government was partially responsible for a lack of transparency that has marred the response to the fast-expanding health crisis."

Canada reported its first confirmed case and another presumptive case. Health officials have confirmed the fifth case of coronavirus in Australia, and have suspected an additional 5. The Sri Lankan Health Ministry confirms its first case of coronavirus, a 43 year old Chinese woman. Cambodia confirms its first case of the virus, a Chinese man who came with his family to Sihanoukville. Singapore confirms a fifth case, a 56 year old Chinese national who arrived from Wuhan on 18 January. Germany confirmed its first case in Bavaria, a case of domestic transmission. Taiwan reports its first case of domestic transmission of the coronavirus.

Beijing reports first death from coronavirus. Three new suspected cases in Austria; previous suspected cases tested negative. The 'Matei Bals' Institute reported the first possible case in Romania. Ecuador reported a suspected case of coronavirus, a Chinese citizen who arrived from Hong Kong. Fiji authorities are holding six Chinese travelers in quarantine in Nadi as a precaution after they failed to gain entry to Samoa due to Samoa's quarantine requirements that were implemented Friday. The quarantine requirements, imposed after an emergency Cabinet meeting, compel anyone who's been in China to "self-quarantine" in a country free from the coronavirus for 14 days. In Poland, two children were admitted to the Kraków hospital with the suspicion of coronavirus. In Mongolia a 14-year-old girl who was studying in China had fallen ill with a suspected case of pneumonia and laryngitis; she was pronounced dead on the same day. Health authorities have since taken a sample from the deceased girl to be analysed at the National Center for Communicable Diseases in Ulaanbaatar. Two Mongolian students returning from Taiwan to Chinggis Khaan International Airport have shown symptoms of high fever and rising temperature and were put into quarantine after landing in Mongolia. In Switzerland, two people were put under quarantine at the Triemli Hospital in Zurich, both had previously been to China. These cases later turned up negative.

In Germany, the first specific, global case of coronavirus being transmitted by a person with no symptoms has been reported. The originally-infected individual is from Shanghai.

28 January

China's Supreme People's Court ruled that whistleblower, Li Wenliang, had not committed the crime of spreading "rumors" when on 30 December 2019 he posted to a WeChat forum for medical school alumni that seven patients under his care appeared to have contracted SARS. In their ruling, the Supreme People's Court stated, "If society had at the time believed those 'rumours', and wore masks, used disinfectant and avoided going to the wildlife market as if there were a SARS outbreak, perhaps it would've meant we could better control the coronavirus today," the court said. "Rumours end when there is openness."

WHO Situation Report 8: Thailand confirms six more cases, bringing the total infected there to 14. Thailand's health minister, Anutin Charnvirakul, states that "we are not able to stop the spread" of coronavirus in the country. Singapore confirms two more cases, bringing the total infected in Singapore to seven. That was followed by a Hubei-related suspension from 29 January. Japan confirms 3 additional cases, bringing the total infected in Japan to seven, including a man who had never visited Wuhan. He was working as a tour bus driver and had driven a group from Wuhan earlier in January. Germany's first confirmed case, reported the previous day, had occurred in a German citizen who had not travelled to China. However, he had close contact with a visiting Chinese colleague who reported starting to feel ill during her return flight to Shanghai and she was diagnosed with coronavirus infection after arriving in China. Germany confirmed 3 new cases, all of whom were coworkers of the first confirmed patient. France confirmed its fourth case, an elderly Chinese tourist who is in critical condition.

The Brazilian Ministry of Health reports three suspected cases ongoing in three locations: Belo Horizonte (MG), Curitiba (PR) and São Leopoldo (RS). Canada reports a new presumptive case in British Columbia, a man in his 40s who had recently travelled to Wuhan.

A UK-Chinese medical research paper reports a statistical model finding that "estimates suggest the actual number of infected cases could be much higher than the reported, with estimated 26,701 cases (as of 28th January 2020)." Scientists from The Peter Doherty Institute for Infection and Immunity (Doherty Institute) in Melbourne reported that they had successfully grown 2019-nCoV from a patient sample.

Xiangyang became quarantined starting 00:00; the entire Hubei province thus became quarantined save for Shennongjia Forestry District.

29 January

WHO Situation Report 9: Tibet reported its first suspected case identified on the previous day and declared a level 1 health emergency in the evening, the last mainland provincial division to do so. Suspected cases have now been reported in all 31 mainland provincial divisions.

Companies in Hubei are required not to resume services before 13 February, and schools in Hubei are to postpone the reopening of schools.

The UAE confirms its first case. Shortly afterwards, an Emirates' news agency confirmed four people from a Chinese family to be infected. Finland reports its first case of the virus in Lapland, found in a Chinese tourist who left Wuhan before Wuhan was locked down. Singapore confirms three more cases of the virus, bringing the total infected to 10 cases. Malaysia confirms three additional cases, bringing its total to seven. Japan reports four additional cases, including a tour bus guide that was on the same bus as one of the cases confirmed on 28 January and three evacuated from Wuhan. France confirmed a 5th case, the daughter of the patient in the fourth case.

Two Chinese nationals were placed in isolation wards in Armenia amid the first suspected case of coronavirus in the country. The Chinese nationals were tourists travelling to Armenia from neighbouring Georgia. Liana Torosyan, the head of the Department of Infectious Diseases, advised that samples will be sent to European labs, as Armenia does not have the capacity to test for the novel coronavirus. Brazil reports a total of 9 suspected cases in six states of the country.

Air Canada is halting all direct flights to China following the federal government's advisory to avoid non-essential travel to the mainland due to the coronavirus epidemic. The suspension is effective Thursday and slated to last until Feb. 29.

30 January

WHO Situation Report 10: Tibet confirms its first case, which was previously suspected. Cases have now been confirmed in all 31 provincial divisions of mainland China. India confirms its first case of coronavirus in a student who had returned from Wuhan University to the Indian state of Kerala. Philippines confirms its first case of coronavirus in a female Chinese national who arrived in Manila via Hong Kong on 21 January. Japan confirms three more cases, bringing the total to 14. Malaysia confirms one more case, bringing the total to eight. Singapore confirms three more cases, bringing the total to 13. South Korea confirms two more cases, with one of them being the first human-to-human transmission there. Vietnam confirms three new cases, bringing the total to five. France confirms its sixth case. Italy confirms its first two cases in a press conference by the Prime Minister, Giuseppe Conte. Germany confirms its fifth case, an employee of the company where the four previously known cases are also employed.

The United States confirmed its sixth case, the spouse of another patient in Chicago. This is the first confirmed case of human to human transmission within the United States.

31 January

WHO Situation Report 11: The United Kingdom and Russia confirmed their first coronavirus infections. First Swedish and Spanish cases were confirmed. Seventh confirmed case in the U.S. is in Santa Clara County, California. A fourth case of coronavirus in Canada has been confirmed in London, Ontario. Thailand confirmed five more cases with the first human-to-human virus transmission inside the country of a local taxi driver, bringing the total to 19. Singapore confirmed three more cases, bringing the total to 16. Chinese health experts warn the public that coronavirus patients can become reinfected. China starts repatriating citizens to Wuhan.

REACTIONS AND MEASURES OUTSIDE MAINLAND CHINA

Running summary (as of 10 February 2020): Aside from China, the 27 nations with 2019-nCoV coronavirus infections are Australia, Belgium, Cambodia, Canada, Finland, France, Germany, Hong Kong, India, Italy, Japan, Macau, Malaysia, Nepal, Philippines, Russia, Singapore, South Korea, Spain, Sri Lanka, Sweden, Taiwan, Thailand, United Arab Emirates, United Kingdom, United States and Vietnam.

Strict surveillance measures are being enforced at airports, seaports and border crossings to prevent the disease wide-spreading into countries/territories which share border or locate in the neighbourhood of the China Mainland. Accordingly, Japan, South Korea, Taiwan and some ASEAN countries (notably Myanmar, the Philippines, Indonesia, Thailand, Singapore, and Vietnam) are thermally monitoring passengers arriving at their major international airports, while flights from and/ or to Wuhan were ceased operating. Activity through gateways in Laos, Myanmar and Vietnam are put under extra supervision from the Government and medical staffs. More seriously, North Korea even bans international flights and foreign visitors, and Papua New Guinea bans travellers from all Asian countries.

Mongolia, North Korea, and Russia have closed their borders with mainland China. Hong Kong closes four out of its eleven border checkpoints with mainland China. Nepal shuts down Rasuwa Fort border crossing for a fortnight. Vietnam shuts down two border gates, with nine auxiliary gates while the others are still in active with strict measures. PNG ordered a close on border with Indonesia on the island of New Guinea. The Inter-Korean Liaison Office was halted for an unspecified time.

Singapore has closed its borders to all recent travellers of China. Vietnam ceased issuing visa to Chinese citizens, only apart from diplomatic work. Kazakhstan, Malaysia, Sri Lanka, the Philippines suspend visa issuance either: on arrival with Chinese citizens, toward the entire infected area of China, toward Hubei-related visitors who previously had travel history or currently hold a passport issued by Hubei and its neighbourhood's authorities.

The United States is closing its borders to all foreign nationals "who pose a threat of transmitting the virus from entering the country and would quarantine U.S. citizens returning from Hubei province in China, the epicentre of the outbreak, for up to 14 days," starting Sunday, 2 February at 5 p.m. This was announced the same day as Singapore's similar action.

3 January

Thailand began screening passengers arriving from Wuhan at four different airports.

Singapore began screening passengers at Changi Airport on the same day.

6 January

The US Centers for Disease Control and Prevention (USCDC) issued a travel watch at Level 1 ("Practice usual precautions") on 6 January, with recommendations on washing hands and more specifically advising avoiding animals, animal markets, and contact with unwell people if travelling to Wuhan.

21 January

The World Health Organization announced that it would hold an emergency meeting on the virus the following day to determine if the virus is a "public health emergency of international concern (PHEIC)".

The Panamanian government has enhanced its sanitary control and screening measures at all ports of entry, in order to prevent the spread of the virus, isolating and testing potential cases.

22 January

North Korea closed its borders and banned foreign tourists over the nCoV. WHO's emergency committee was unable to reach a consensus—with one member stating that the vote was "50/50. Even."—on whether the outbreak should be classified as PHEIC due to lack of information. The committee will resume discussion the next day.

23 January

Following the first laboratory-confirmed case on 23 January, Singaporean airline Scoot cancelled flights to Wuhan between 23 and 26 January over the virus outbreak, after a lockdown was imposed. Schools have also asked parents to declare their travel plans and monitor their children's health. Other measures will also be taken to ensure the safety of students. MINDEF has since issued two medical advisories to service personnel.

Flights in and out of North Korea were halted. Coronavirus cases in Sinuiju were suspected and promptly quarantined for two weeks.

24 January

Following the two laboratory-confirmed cases on 23 January, Vietnam Aviation Authority sent a written directive requesting that all flights from and to Wuhan, to be cancelled immediately until further notice and the tickets should be refunded. Exceptionally, the Authority operates four special flights to carry Wuhan passengers home during the period from 24–27 January, and a backward flight to excavate Vietnamese citizens and diplomats.

Border control measures in Singapore are enhanced and extended to land and sea checkpoints, with the Immigration and Checkpoints Authority and Maritime and Port Authority of Singapore starting temperature checks from noon of that day.

The Russian Far East had closed its border with China until 7 February, while Russian tour operators were inhibited starting 27 January.

25 January

Hong Kong declared a state of emergency and announced it would close schools until 17 February. Hong Kong Disneyland and Ocean Park are closed until further notice.

The United States announced plans to evacuate US citizens out of Wuhan by charter jet. The US government later clarified that it only had limited capacity for private citizen evacuations.

26 January

Hong Kong announced it will ban anyone who has been to Hubei Province in the last 14 days from entering the city starting 27 January.

27 January

Mongolia closed its border with China, shut down schools until 2 March, and called for all public gatherings to be cancelled. The pair of international border gates Hekou (Yunnan, China) - Lào Cai (Vietnam) are suspended against Chinese tourists. The decision was declared by the head of Lào Cai Department of Culture, Sports and Tourism, after an urgent notice from Yunnan Province's Authorities.

The Government of Gilgit Baltistan decided to delay opening the China-Pakistan border crossing point at Khunjerab Pass, scheduled for February.

Following the action from Hong Kong authorities, Macau stated that it will deny entry to visitors from the Mainland's Hubei province or those who had visited the province 14 days prior to arrival unless they are virus-free.

Singapore imposed a 14 days leave of absence for those working in schools, healthcare and eldercare who travelled to China in the last 14 days. Students who returned from these places will do home-based learning instead. In addition, people who went to China the last 14 days must fill health and travel declarations and monitor health with temperature checks.

Malaysia suspends all visa facilities for Chinese tourists from Hubei and its neighbouring provinces in China.

Tijuana, Mexico receives its final scheduled non-stop flight from mainland China before a previously scheduled suspension of service. Passengers and crew were screened by health officials upon arrival to the Tijuana International Airport. Flights between Tijuana and Mainland China are scheduled to resume in May 2020.

The USCDC expands travel advisory from Wuhan to the whole of Hubei Province. Later that day, the US State Department raised the travel advisory for China to Level 3 ("Reconsider Travel: Avoid travel due to serious risks to safety and security.")

due to coronavirus. The same day, the USCDC again updates its travel health notice to Warning - Level 3, Avoid All Nonessential Travel to China.

28 January

The Philippines and Sri Lanka suspended issuance of visa-on-arrival to Chinese nationals.

Singapore announced a suspension from 29 January, 12 pm of entry or transit for all new visitors with recent Hubei travel history within the last 14 days, or holders of China passports issued in Hubei. Hong Kong temporarily closes four of the eleven ports with the Mainland. Carrie Lam, the Chief Executive, stated the high-speed rail service between Hong Kong and mainland China would be suspended starting 30 January and all cross-border ferry services would also be suspended in a bid to stop the spread of coronavirus. Additionally, flights from mainland China would be cut in half, cross-border bus services reduced, and the Hong Kong government is asking all its employees (except those providing essential or emergency services) to work from home. In a later press conference, Carrie Lam said that the Man Kam To and Sha Tau Kok border checkpoints would be closed.

Thailand starts scanning all travellers from China with immediate effect.

The UK's Foreign Office warns Britons not to travel to mainland China, unless their journey is essential.

The USCDC stated it was boosting staffing at 20 US airports that have quarantine facilities.

29 January

The Government of Papua New Guinea bans all travellers from Asian countries and shut down its border with Indonesia. The order takes effect from 30 January.

Palau and Vanuatu temporarily suspended flights from mainland China, Macau, and Hong Kong until the end of February and restricted diplomatic work in those destinations. Federated States of Micronesia is considering the same measures.

The Government of Kazakhstan suspended visa issuance to Chinese citizens. In addition, all transport links from and to China have been halted; accordingly, movement by train will stop on 1 February, by airplane will stop from 3 February. Georgia temporarily suspended all direct flights with China.

Rasuwa Fort, which is a border crossing between Rasuwa District (Nepal) and Tibet (China), will be sealed for 15 days starting 29 January. The decision was preceded by a meeting between security and immigration authorities of two countries earlier that day.

The WHO announces that its director-general has decided to reconvene their international health regulations emergency committee on 30 January to reconsider declaring a global health emergency, technically a "public health emergency of international concern" (PHEIC). The reconvening is due "mainly on the evidence of increasing number of cases, human-to-human transmission outside of China, and the further development of transmission." The committee meeting is planned to start at 13:30 Geneva time. Further, the WHO announces their having set up "The Pandemic Supply Chain Network (PSCN)" in collaboration with the World Economic Forum.

The Government of Canada issued a travel advisory to avoid non-essential travel to China due to the novel coronavirus outbreak. The Government of Canada also issued a regional travel advisory to avoid all travel to the Province of Hubei— including the cities of Wuhan, Huanggang and Ezhou—due to the imposition of heavy travel restrictions in order to limit the spread of the novel coronavirus. On the same day, the Minister of Foreign Affairs François-Philippe Champagne announced that an aircraft would be sent to repatriate Canadians from the areas affected by the novel coronavirus in China. As a result of the travel advisories issued by the Canadian government, Air Canada suspended all direct flights to China until at least 29 February.

The Ministry of Popular Power for Health announced that the Rafael Rangel National Institute of Hygiene (Spanish: *Instituto Nacional de Higiene Rafael Rangel*) in Caracas will perform the detection of other respiratory viruses based on non-influenza types, including coronaviruses in humans. It is also the only health institute in the country with installed capacity for the diagnosis of respiratory viruses in Venezuela and is able carry out logistics in the 23 states, the Capital District and Federal Dependencies.

British Airways and Lufthansa cancel all flights to and from mainland China.

Singapore expands temperature screening to cover all incoming flights with additional checks on flights from China and passengers from Hubei.

30 January

Vietnam shuts down air traffic with China. The Ministry of Public Security temporarily ceased issuing visa to Chinese citizens within the epidemic areas. Additionally, crossing at gateways, airports, seaports are put under higher supervision, with strict monitoring and medical check-ups (applied to both humans and items; prohibited against wildlife animals and derivatives). Later that day, after confirmation of the first three Vietnamese patients, the Prime Minister ordered: further visa restriction only apart from diplomatic work, suspension of activities at border gates (with China) where are still in active, excavation for citizens when necessary, and an emergency alert being considered.

The Liaison Office between two Koreas in the border town of Kaesong was shut down for an unspecified time regarding infection concern. The decision was made after negotiations between the representatives of both countries earlier morning on 30 January, informed by the Unification Ministry of South Korea.

North Korea's news agency KCNA declared a "state emergency" and reported the establishment of anti-epidemic headquarters around the country.

Singapore announced that every household was to receive four masks starting from 1 February.

Russia announces restrictions on railway travel with China, such that only a direct train between Moscow and Beijing remains.

The WHO director-general declares the coronavirus outbreak a "Public Health Emergency of International Concern" (PHEIC), reversing two previous decisions after emergency committee meetings in the last week.

Italian Prime Minister Giuseppe Conte stated in a press conference that Italy had closed all air traffic to and from China. It is believed that Conte has also called a cabinet meeting for Friday to discuss further actions. Six thousand people are briefly quarantined on board an Italian cruise ship as tests are carried out on two Chinese passengers suspected of having coronavirus, a spokesman for the Costa Crociere cruise company said. The same day, all passengers are released as it is found that the ill individual has the flu, not coronavirus.

The US State Department issued an updated travel advisory as "Level 4: Do Not Travel to China." Its website stated that "Those currently in China should consider departing" and warning that "Travelers should be prepared for travel restrictions to be put into effect with little or no advance notice". Additionally, it authorized American diplomatic staff and their families to evacuate China. The State of Washington in the US declared a Level 1 Emergency and activated its Emergency Response Center for dealing with the now global coronavirus outbreak.

British foreign secretary Dominic Raab disclosed that the emergency flight containing about 120 Britons from Wuhan that was delayed by 24 hours, was due to land at RAF Brize Norton on Friday morning, where the passengers will be taken to Wirral for a fortnight's quarantine.

Trinidad and Tobago's health minister, Terrance Deyalsingh, announced that Trinidad & Tobago had decided to implement restrictions on persons travelling from China. Persons who are living or who have visited China, will be barred from entering Trinidad & Tobago unless they had already been out of China 14 days prior to attempting to travel to Trinidad & Tobago.

Air France and KLM cancel all flights to mainland China until February 9.

31 January

Russian authorities announced the border closure with China would be extended to at least 1 March.

Singapore closes borders to all visitors arriving from mainland China (including passengers transiting through Singapore) except Singaporeans, Singapore residents and long-term visa holders. Macau announced it would postpone schools indefinitely and that schools should contact students to arrange for assignments to be done online. Hong Kong extends public holiday to the 2nd of March, and also requests all visitors who have been in Hubei in the past 14 days to be quarantined. All government employees may work at their own home until the 9th of February.

Italy declared a state of emergency, the first EU country to do so, and allocates an initial 5 million Euros to tackle the virus.

The United States government declares a Public Health Emergency due to the coronavirus, and is closing its borders to all foreign nationals "who pose a threat of transmitting the virus from entering the country and would quarantine U.S. citizens returning from Hubei province in China, the epicenter of the outbreak, for up to 14 days," starting Sunday, Feb. 2 at 5 p.m. The 195 Americans on the Air Force base in California whom were recently evacuated from Wuhan recently shall also be quarantined.

Jamaica's health minister, Christopher Tufton, announced that a government decision to ban travel between China and Jamaica. All persons entering Jamaica from China will be subject to immediate quarantine for at least 14 days, and anyone who was allowed to land and shows symptoms of the virus will be put in immediate isolation. In keeping with the new policy, 19 Chinese nationals who arrived at the Norman Manley International Airport on the evening of 31 January were denied entry, quarantined and put on a flight back to China on 1 February.

The Ministry of Health, Catalina Andramuño, announced that the country now possess reactives for testing new cases locally, becoming the first in South America.

LOT Polish Airlines cancels all flights to Beijing until 9 February. Delta Airlines suspends all China flights, and American Airlines pilots sue for same action. Later, American Airlines ceased flights to China as well. Later still, United Airlines halts all flights to China, excepting San Francisco to Hong Kong.

Basra International Airport in Iraq has declared that passengers of any nationality travelling from China will be denied entry.

Turkish Airlines halted all flights to China until 9 February.

2020 HUBEI LOCKDOWNS

On 23 January 2020, the central government of the People's Republic of China imposed a lockdown in Wuhan and other cities in Hubei province in an effort to quarantine the epicentre of an outbreak of coronavirus disease 2019 (COVID-19). This was the first known instance in modern history of locking down a major city of as many as 11 million people, and the incident was commonly referred to in the media as the "Wuhan lockdown". The World Health Organization (WHO), although stating that it was beyond its own guidelines, commended the move, calling it "unprecedented in public health history". The lockdown in Wuhan set the precedence for similar measures in other Chinese cities. Within hours of the Wuhan lockdown, travel restrictions were also imposed on the nearby cities of Huanggang and Ezhou, and were eventually imposed on all 15 other cities in Hubei, affecting a total of about 57 million people. On 2 February 2020, Wenzhou, Zhejiang, implemented a seven-day lockdown in which only one person per household was allowed to exit once each two days, and most of the highway exits were closed.

Background

Wuhan is the capital of Hubei province in China. With a population of over 11 million, it is the largest city in Hubei, the most populous city in Central China, the seventh-most populous Chinese city, and one of the nine National Central Cities of China. Wuhan lies in the eastern Jianghan Plain, on the confluence of the Yangtze River and its largest tributary, the Han River. It is a major transportation hub, with dozens of railways, roads and expressways passing through the city and connecting to other major cities. Because of its key role in domestic transport, Wuhan is known as the "Nine Provinces' Thoroughfare" and sometimes referred to as "the Chicago of China".

Lockdowns

Hubei

In mid-December 2019, an emerging cluster of people, many linked to the Huanan Seafood Wholesale Market in Wuhan, were infected with pneumonia with no clear causes. Chinese scientists subsequently linked the pneumonia to a new strain of coronavirus that was given the initial designation SARS-CoV-2.

On 10 January 2020, the first death and 41 clinically confirmed infections caused by the coronavirus were reported.

By 22 January 2020, the novel coronavirus had spread to major cities and provinces in China, with 571 confirmed cases and 17 deaths reported. Confirmed cases were also reported in other regions and countries, including Hong Kong, Macau, Taiwan, Thailand, Japan, South Korea, and the United States.

At 2 am on 23 January 2020, authorities issued a notice informing residents of Wuhan that from 10am, all public transport, including buses, railways, flights, and ferry services would be suspended. The Wuhan Airport, the Wuhan railway station, and the Wuhan metro were all closed. The residents of Wuhan were also not allowed to leave the city without permission from the authorities. The notice caused an exodus from Wuhan. An estimated 300,000 people were reported to have left Wuhan by train alone before the 10 am lockdown. By the afternoon of 23 January, the authorities began shutting down some of the major highways leaving Wuhan. The lockdown came two days before the Chinese New Year, the most important festival in the country, and traditionally the peak traveling season, when millions of Chinese travel across the country.

Following the lockdown of Wuhan, public transportation systems in two of Wuhan's neighboring prefecture-level cities, Huanggang and Ezhou, were also placed on lockdown. A total of 12 other county to prefecture-level cities in Hubei, including Huangshi, Jingzhou, Yichang, Xiaogan, Jingmen, Suizhou, Xianning, Qianjiang, Xiantao, Shiyan, Tianmen and Enshi, were placed on traveling restrictions by the end of 24 January, bringing the number of people affected by the restriction to more than 50 million.

Elsewhere in China

On 2 February 2020, Wenzhou, Zhejiang, implemented a 7-day restriction where each household was only allowed to have one person leave their home for provisions every two days. This was the first lockdown outside of the Hubei province. 46 of the 54 highway exits in Wenzhou were also closed, effectively placing the city of about 9 million in a semi-lockdown.

Impacts and reactions

The exodus from Wuhan before the lockdown has resulted in angry responses on Sina Weibo from residents in other cities who are concerned that it could result in spreading of the novel coronavirus to their cities. Some in Wuhan are concerned with the availability of provisions and especially medical supplies during the lockdown.

The World Health Organization called the Wuhan lockdown "unprecedented" and said it showed "how committed the authorities are to contain a viral breakout". However, WHO clarified that the move is not a recommendation that WHO had made and authorities have to wait and see how effective it is. The WHO has separately stated that the possibility of locking down an entire city like this is "new to science".

The CSI 300 Index, an aggregate measure of the top 300 stocks in the Shanghai and Shenzhen stock exchanges, dropped almost 3% on 23 January 2020, the biggest single-day loss in almost 9 months, after the Wuhan lockdown was announced as investors spooked by the drastic measure sought safe haven for their investments.

The unprecedented scale of this lockdown generated controversy, and at least one expert criticized this measure as "risky business" that "could very easily backfire" by forcing otherwise healthy people in Wuhan to stay in close conditions with infected people. Drawing a cordon sanitaire around a city of 11 million people raises inevitable ethical concerns. It also drew comparisons to the lockdown of the poor West Point neighbourhood in Liberia during the 2014 ebola outbreak, which was lifted after ten days.

The lockdown has caused panic in the city of Wuhan, and many have expressed concern about the city's ability to cope with the outbreak. It remains unknown whether the large costs of this measure, both financially and in terms of personal liberty, will translate to effective infection control.

Medical historian Howard Markel argued that the Chinese government "may now be overreacting, imposing an unjustifiable burden on the population," and that "Incremental restrictions, enforced steadily and transparently, tend to work far better than draconian measures."

WORLD EXPERTS AND FUNDERS SET PRIORITIES FOR COVID-19 RESEARCH

Leading health experts from around the world have been meeting at the World Health Organization's Geneva headquarters to assess the current level of knowledge about the new COVID-19 disease, identify gaps and work together to accelerate and fund priority research needed to help stop this outbreak and prepare for any future outbreaks.

The 2-day forum was convened in line with the WHO R&D Blueprint – a strategy for developing drugs and vaccines before epidemics, and accelerating research and development while they are occurring.

"This outbreak is a test of solidarity — political, financial and scientific. We need to come together to fight a common enemy that does not respect borders, ensure that we have the resources necessary to bring this outbreak to an end and bring our best science to the forefront to find shared answers to shared problems. Research is an integral part of the outbreak response," said WHO Director-General

Dr Tedros Adhanom Ghebreyesus. "I appreciate the positive response of the research community to join us at short notice and come up with concrete plans and commitment to work together."

The meeting, hosted in collaboration with GloPID-R (the Global Research Collaboration for Infectious Disease Preparedness) brought together major research funders and over 300 scientists and researchers from a large variety of disciplines. They discussed all aspects of the outbreak and ways to control it including:

- the natural history of the virus, its transmission and diagnosis;
- animal and environmental research on the origin of the virus, including management measures at the human-animal interface;
- epidemiological studies;
- clinical characterization and management of disease caused by the virus;
- infection prevention and control, including best ways to protect health care workers;
- research and development for candidate therapeutics and vaccines;
- ethical considerations for research;
- and integration of social sciences into the outbreak response.

"This meeting allowed us to identify the urgent priorities for research. As a group of funders we will continue to mobilize, coordinate and align our funding to enable the research needed to tackle this crisis and stop the outbreak, in partnership with WHO," said Professor Yazdan Yazdanpanah, chair of GloPID-R. "Equitable access – making sure we share data and reach those most in need, in particular those in lower and middle-income countries, is fundamental to this work which must be guided by ethical considerations at all times."

During the meeting, the more than 300 scientists and researchers participating both in person and virtually agreed on a set of global research priorities. They also outlined mechanisms for continuing scientific interactions and collaborations beyond the meeting which will be coordinated and facilitated by WHO. They worked with research funders to determine how necessary resources can be mobilized so that critical research can start immediately.

The deliberations will form the basis of a research and innovation roadmap charting all the research needed and this will be used by researchers and funders to accelerate the research response.

A NOVEL CORONAVIRUS FROM PATIENTS WITH PNEUMONIA IN CHINA

In late December 2019, several local health facilities reported clusters of patients with pneumonia of unknown cause that were epidemiologically linked to a seafood and wet animal wholesale market in Wuhan, Hubei Province, China. On December 31, 2019, the Chinese Center for Disease Control and Prevention (China CDC) dispatched a rapid response team to accompany Hubei provincial and Wuhan city health authorities and to conduct an epidemiologic and etiologic investigation. We report the results of this investigation, identifying the source of the pneumonia clusters, and describe a novel coronavirus detected in patients with pneumonia whose specimens were tested by the China CDC at an early stage of the outbreak. We also describe clinical features of the pneumonia in two of these patients.

VIRAL DIAGNOSTIC METHODS

Four lower respiratory tract samples, including bronchoalveolar-lavage fluid, were collected from patients with pneumonia of unknown cause who were identified in Wuhan on December 21, 2019, or later and who had been present at the Huanan Seafood Market close to the time of their clinical presentation. Seven bronchoalveolar-lavage fluid specimens were collected from patients in Beijing hospitals with pneumonia of known cause to serve as control samples. Extraction of nucleic acids from clinical samples (including uninfected cultures that served as negative controls) was performed with a High Pure Viral Nucleic Acid Kit, as described by the manufacturer (Roche).

ISOLATION OF VIRUS

Bronchoalveolar-lavage fluid samples were collected in sterile cups to which virus transport medium was added. Samples were then centrifuged to remove cellular debris. The supernatant was inoculated on human airway epithelial cells, which had been obtained from airway specimens resected from patients undergoing surgery for lung cancer and were confirmed to be special-pathogen-free by NGS.

Human airway epithelial cells were expanded on plastic substrate to generate passage-1 cells and were subsequently plated at a density of $2.5×10^5$ cells per well on permeable Transwell-COL (12-mm diameter) supports. Human airway epithelial cell cultures were generated in an air–liquid interface for 4 to 6 weeks to form well-differentiated, polarized cultures resembling in vivo pseudostratified mucociliary epithelium.

Prior to infection, apical surfaces of the human airway epithelial cells were washed three times with phosphate-buffered saline; 150 ìl of supernatant from bronchoalveolar-lavage fluid samples was inoculated onto the apical surface of the cell cultures. After a 2-hour incubation at 37°C, unbound virus was removed by washing with 500 ìl of phosphate-buffered saline for 10 minutes; human airway epithelial cells were maintained in an airliquid interface incubated at 37°C with 5% carbon dioxide.

Every 48 hours, 150 ìl of phosphate-buffered saline was applied to the apical surfaces of the human airway epithelial cells, and after 10 minutes of incubation at 37°C the samples were harvested. Pseudostratified mucociliary epithelium cells were maintained in this environment; apical samples were passaged in a 1:3 diluted vial stock to new cells. The cells were monitored daily with light microscopy, for cytopathic effects, and with RT-PCR, for the presence of viral nucleic acid in the supernatant. After three passages, apical samples and human airway epithelial cells were prepared for transmission electron microscopy.

TRANSMISSION ELECTRON MICROSCOPY

Supernatant from human airway epithelial cell cultures that showed cytopathic effects was collected, inactivated with 2% paraformaldehyde for at least 2 hours, and ultracentrifuged to sediment virus particles.

The enriched supernatant was negatively stained on film-coated grids for examination. Human airway epithelial cells showing cytopathic effects were collected and fixed with 2% paraformaldehyde–2.5% glutaraldehyde and were then fixed with 1% osmium tetroxide dehydrated with grade ethanol embedded with PON812 resin. Sections (80 nm) were cut from resin block and stained with uranyl acetate and lead citrate, separately. The negative stained grids and ultrathin sections were observed under transmission electron microscopy.

VIRAL GENOME SEQUENCING

RNA extracted from bronchoalveolar-lavage fluid and culture supernatants was used as a template to clone and sequence the genome. We used a combination of Illumina sequencing and nanopore sequencing to characterize the virus genome.

Sequence reads were assembled into contig maps (a set of overlapping DNA segments) with the use of CLC Genomics software, version 4.6.1 (CLC Bio). Specific primers were subsequently designed for PCR, and 52- or 32-RACE (rapid amplification of cDNA ends) was used to fill genome gaps from conventional Sanger sequencing. These PCR products were purified from gels and sequenced with a BigDye Terminator v3.1 Cycle Sequencing Kit and a 3130XL Genetic Analyzer, in accordance with the manufacturers' instructions.

Multiple-sequence alignment of the 2019-nCoV and reference sequences was performed with the use of Muscle. Phylogenetic analysis of the complete genomes was performed with RA × ML (13) with 1000 bootstrap replicates and a general time-reversible model used as the nucleotide substitution model.

DETECTION AND ISOLATION OF A NOVEL CORONAVIRUS

Three bronchoalveolar-lavage samples were collected from Wuhan Jinyintan Hospital on December 30, 2019. No specific pathogens (including HCoV-229E, HCoV-NL63, HCoV-OC43, and HCoV-HKU1) were detected in clinical specimens from these patients by the RespiFinderSmart22kit. RNA extracted from bronchoalveolar-lavage fluid from the patients was used as a template to clone and sequence a genome using a combination of Illumina sequencing and nanopore sequencing. More than 20,000 viral reads from individual specimens were obtained, and most contigs matched to the genome from lineage B of the genus betacoronavirus — showing more than 85% identity with a bat SARS-like CoV (bat-SL-CoVZC45, MG772933.1) genome published previously. Positive results were also obtained with use of a real-time RT-PCR assay for RNA targeting to a consensus RdRp region of pan â-CoV (although the cycle threshold value was higher than 34 for detected samples).

Virus isolation from the clinical specimens was performed with human airway epithelial cells and Vero E6 and Huh-7 cell lines. The isolated virus was named 2019-nCoV.

To determine whether virus particles could be visualized in 2019-nCoV–infected human airway epithelial cells, mock-infected and 2019-nCoV–infected human airway epithelial cultures were examined with light microscopy daily and with transmission electron microscopy 6 days after inoculation. Cytopathic effects were observed 96 hours after inoculation on surface layers of human airway epithelial cells; a lack of cilium beating was seen with light microcopy in the center of the focus. No specific cytopathic effects were observed in the Vero E6 and Huh-7 cell lines until 6 days after inoculation.

Electron micrographs of negative-stained 2019-nCoV particles were generally spherical with some pleomorphism. Diameter varied from about 60 to 140 nm. Virus particles had quite distinctive spikes, about 9 to 12 nm, and gave virions the appearance of a solar corona. Extracellular free virus particles and inclusion bodies filled with virus particles in membrane-bound vesicles in cytoplasm were found in the human airway epithelial ultrathin sections. This observed morphology is consistent with the Coronaviridae family.

To further characterize the virus, de novo sequences of 2019-nCoV genome from clinical specimens (bronchoalveolar-lavage fluid) and human airway epithelial cell virus isolates were obtained by Illumina and nanopore sequencing. The novel coronavirus was identified from all three patients.

Although 2019-nCoV is similar to some betacoronaviruses detected in bats, it is distinct from SARS-CoV and MERS-CoV. The three 2019-nCoV coronaviruses from Wuhan, together with two bat-derived SARS-like strains, ZC45 and ZXC21, form a distinct clade. SARS-CoV strains from humans and genetically similar SARS-like coronaviruses from bats collected from southwestern China formed another clade within the subgenus sarbecovirus. Since the sequence identity in conserved replicase domains (ORF 1ab) is less than 90% between 2019-nCoV and other members of betacoronavirus, the 2019-nCoV — the likely causative agent of the viral pneumonia in Wuhan — is a novel betacoronavirus belonging to the sarbecovirus subgenus of Coronaviridae family.

CORONAVIRUS QUARANTINE IN WUHAN

Wuhan plans to round up those suspected of having the virus to be placed in isolation, in some kind of mass quarantine camps, The New York Times reported. China's Vice Premier Sun Chunlan said that city officials should go door to door to check residents' temperatures and to interview those in contact with infected individuals, the Times reported.

"Set up a 24-hour duty system. During these wartime conditions, there must be no deserters, or they will be nailed to the pillar of historical shame forever," Sun said, according to the Times.

The Times is reporting a shortage of medical supplies, coronavirus-testing kits and hospital beds due to the lockdown in the city and surrounding area, leading to people walking on foot from hospital to hospital, only to be turned away.

Who will be quarantined in the US?

Officials announced on Friday (Jan. 31) that the U.S. will be enforcing quarantines on citizens who have traveled to the Hubei Province (where the outbreak originated) in the last 14 days. If U.S. citizens have been to China in the last 14 days, they will be rerouted to one of eleven airports across the country to be screened for the new coronavirus, according to the Department of Homeland Security (DHS).

If passengers who have traveled to China are showing symptoms of the virus (which include a cough, trouble breathing or fever) they will be subject to mandatory quarantines. If passengers who have traveled to China (outside of the Hubei province) show no symptoms after being screened at one of the 11 airports, they will be re-booked to their destinations within the U.S. and asked to self-quarantine at home, according to the DHS.

Other travelers who haven't been to China but are found to be on the same flight of passengers that have been to China might also be rerouted to one of the 11 airports, according to the DHS. What's more, in general "foreign nationals" who have traveled to China in the past 14 days won't be allowed in the U.S.

Hundreds of U.S. citizens who were evacuated from Wuhan are currently under mandatory quarantine at several U.S. military bases.

Does the coronavirus have an official name?

On Feb. 11, WHO Director-General Tedros Adhanom Ghebreyesus announced the official name of the new disease caused by the novel coronavirus: Corona Virus Disease, abbreviated as COVID-19. "Having a name matters to prevent the use of other names that can be inaccurate or stigmatizing. It also gives us a standard format to use for any future coronavirus outbreaks," Ghebreyesus said. WHO discourages naming new viruses after geographic locations, people, species or classes of animals or foods, according to the organization's Best Practices for the Naming of New Human Infectious Diseases.

Rather, WHO encourages use of descriptive terms of a disease, such as "respiratory disease" and "neurologic syndrome," as well as "severe" or "progressive." The organization also says that if a pathogen is known, it should be used as part of the disease's name.

The International Committee on Taxonomy of Viruses is tasked with giving the virus an official name. On Feb. 11, the committee said the virus will be known as "severe acute respiratory syndrome coronavirus 2," or SARS-CoV-2, due to its genetic similarity to the virus that causes severe acute respiratory syndrome (SARS), according to Science Magazine.

What is a coronavirus?

Coronaviruses are a large family of viruses that can cause respiratory illnesses such as the common cold, according to the Centers for Disease Control and Prevention (CDC). Most people get infected with coronaviruses at one point in their lives, but symptoms are typically mild to moderate. In some cases, the viruses can cause lower-respiratory tract illnesses such as pneumonia and bronchitis.

These viruses are common amongst animals worldwide, but only a handful of them are known to affect humans. Rarely, coronaviruses can evolve and spread from animals to humans. This is what happened with the coronaviruses known as the Middle East respiratory syndrome coronavirus (MERS-CoV) and the severe acute respiratory syndrome coronavirus (SARS-Cov), both of which are known to cause more severe symptoms.

Where did the new coronavirus come from? Since the virus first popped up in

Wuhan in people who had visited a local seafood and animal market (called the Huanan seafood market), officials could only say it likely hopped from an animal to humans. In a new study, however, the researchers compared SARS-CoV-2 (formerly 2019-nCoV) genetic sequence with those in a library of viral sequences, and found that the most closely related viruses were two coronaviruses that originated in bats; both of those coronaviruses shared 88% of their genetic sequence with that of SARS-CoV-2.

Based on these results, the authors said the SARS-CoV-2 likely originated in bats. However, no bats were sold at the Huanan seafood market, which suggests that another yet-to-be-identified animal acted as a steppingstone of sorts to transmit the virus to humans.

A previous study suggested snakes, which were sold at the Huanan seafood market, as a possible source of the new virus. However, some experts have criticized the study, saying it's unclear if coronaviruses can infect snakes.

How does the coronavirus spread between people? Researchers are still working to understand exactly how SARS-CoV-2 spreads. But in general, the the most common way coronaviruses spread is through respiratory droplets produced from coughs and sneezes, according to the CDC. Tests have also found the virus present in patients' stool, suggesting it may be able to spread through fecal contamination. However, it is still unclear whether people can catch the virus by touching contaminated surfaces, the CDC says.

Deaths from coronavirus outside China

As of Feb. 13, there have been three reported deaths from the new coronavirus outside of China. These include the deaths of a 44-year-old man in the Philippines, a 39-year-old man in Hong Kong, and a woman in her 80s in Japan.

Could this virus cause a pandemic? In order for this virus, or any, to lead to a pandemic in humans, it needs to do three things: efficiently infect humans, replicate in humans and then spread *easily* among humans, Live Science previously reported. Right now, its unclear how easily the virus spreads from person to person.

To determine how easily the virus spreads, scientists will need to calculate what's known as the "basic reproduction number, or R_0 (pronounced R-nought.) This is an estimate of the average number of people who catch the virus from a single infected person, Live science previously reported.

A study published Jan. 29 in the New England Journal of Medicine (NEJM) estimated an R_0 value for the new coronavirus to be 2.2, meaning each infected person has been spreading the virus to an average of 2.2 people. This is similar to previous estimates, which have placed the R_0 value between 2 and 3. (For comparison, SARS initially had an R_0 of around 3, before public health measures brought it down to less than 1.)

In general, a virus will continue to spread if it has an R value of greater than 1, and so public health measures to stem the outbreak should aim to reduce R_0 to less than one, the authors of the NEJM paper said.

On Jan. 30, the World Health Organization (WHO) declared that the new coronavirus outbreak is a public health emergency of international concern. The main reason for the declaration is concern that the virus could spread to countries with weaker health systems, WHO said.

How does coronavirus compare to SARS and MERS? As of Feb. 9, more people had died from the new coronavirus than from SARS — which killed 774 individuals worldwide, according to The New York Times.

MERS and SARS have both been known to cause severe symptoms in people. It's unclear how the new coronavirus will compare in severity, as it has caused severe symptoms and death in some patients while causing only mild illness in others, according to the CDC. All three of the coronaviruses can be transmitted between humans through close contact. MERS, which was transmitted from touching infected camels or consuming their meat or milk, was first reported in 2012 in Saudi Arabia and has mostly been contained in the Arabian Peninsula, according to NPR. SARS was first reported in 2002 in southern China (no new cases have been reported since 2004) and is thought to have spread from bats that infected civets. The new coronavirus was likely transmitted from touching or eating an infected animal in Wuhan.

During the SARS outbreak, the virus killed about 1 in 10 people who were infected. The death rate from COVID-19 isn't yet known. In the beginning of an outbreak, the initial cases that are identified "skew to the severe," which may make the mortality rate seem higher than it is, Alex Azar, secretary of the U.S. Department of Health and Homeland Security (HHS), said during a news briefing on Tuesday (Jan. 28). The mortality rate may drop as more mild cases are identified, Azar said.

Currently, most of the patients who have died from the infection have been older than 60 and have had preexisting conditions.

What are the symptoms of the new coronavirus and how do you treat it? Symptoms of the new coronavirus include fever, cough and difficulty breathing, according to the CDC. It's estimated that symptoms may appear as soon as two days or as long as 14 days after exposure, the CDC said. The NEJM study published on Jan. 29 estimated that, on average, people show symptoms about five days after they are infected.

There are no specific treatments for coronavirus infections and most people will recover on their own, according to the CDC. So treatment involves rest and medication to relieve symptoms. A humidifier or hot shower can help to relieve a sore throat and cough. If you are mildly sick, you should drink a lot of fluids and rest but if you are worried about your symptoms, you should see a healthcare provider, they wrote. (This is advice for all coronaviruses, not specifically aimed toward the new virus).

There is no vaccine for the new coronavirus, but researchers at the U.S. National Institutes of Health confirmed they were in preliminary stages of developing one. Officials plan to launch a phase 1 clinical trial of a potential vaccine within the next three months, Dr. Anthony Fauci, Director of the National Institute of Allergy and Infectious Diseases, said in a news conference on Jan. 28.

Researchers are also working on gathering samples of the virus to design a therapy that will train patients' immune cells to detect and destroy the virus, Facui said.

How can people protect themselves and others? The best way to prevent infection with COVID-19 is to avoid being exposed to the virus, according to the CDC. In general, the CDC recommends the following to prevent the spread of respiratory viruses: Wash your hands often with soap and water for at least 20 seconds; avoid touching your eyes, nose, and mouth with unwashed hands; avoid close contact with people who are sick; stay home when you are sick and clean and disinfect frequently touched objects and surfaces.

People who traveled to China and became sick with fever, cough or difficulty breathing within the following two weeks should seek medical care right away, and call ahead to inform medical staff about their recent travel, the CDC said.

The CDC does not recommend face masks for people who are well and without symptoms. The agency does recommend face masks for people who show symptoms of the virus and those taking care of someone sick with the virus (including health care workers).

CHINA CORONAVIRUS OUTBREAK: ALL THE LATEST UPDATES

China had 150 new confirmed coronavirus deaths on Sunday, the National Health Commission announced on Monday, pushing the death toll nationwide to 2,592.

This developed as South Korea reported 161 more cases on Monday, bringing its total number of infections to 763. Officials also confirmed two more deaths of virus patients, bringing the country's death toll to seven.

On Sunday, it raised its disease alert to the highest level after a surge in infections and more deaths.

Meanwhile, Turkey, Pakistan and Armenia closed their borders with Iran on Sunday as the latter reported more coronavirus infections and deaths, prompting neighbouring Afghanistan to also introduce travel restrictions.

At least 152 cases and three deaths were also reported in Italy, prompting emergency measures in Europe.

Here are the latest updates:

China says new coronavirus deaths increase with 150

Mainland China had 150 new confirmed coronavirus deaths on Sunday, the National Health Commission said on Monday, up from 97 the previous day. In a statement, the commission also confirmed 409 new infections during the same period, down from 648 reported a day earlier.

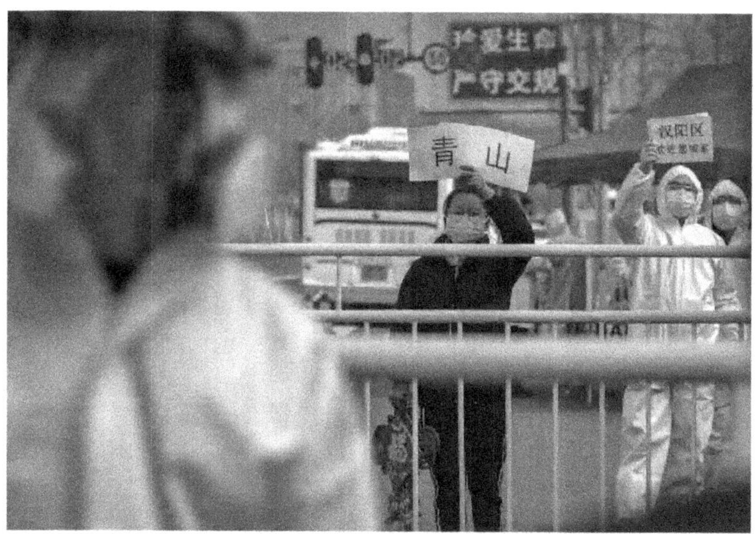

Community workers waiting to pick up recovered coronavirus patients departing from a temporary hospital in Wuhan on Saturday

The total number of confirmed coronavirus cases on the mainland is now 77,150, and 2,592 have died from the outbreak, the commission said.

Meanwhile, China announced that it will allow healthy non-residents of Wuhan to leave the epicentre of the virus.

Four Chinese provinces lower coronavirus emergency response level

Four Chinese provinces; Yunnan, Guangdong, Shanxi and Guizhou, on Monday lowered their coronavirus emergency response measures, local health commissions said. Yunnan and Guizhou cut their emergency response measures from level I to level III, while Guangdong and Shanxi lowered their measures to level II.

China has a four-tier response system for pubic health emergencies that determines what measures it will implement, with level I the most serious. Gansu province was the first to lower its measures on Friday, followed by Liaoning on Saturday.

South Korea reports 161 more coronavirus cases

South Korea reported 161 more cases of the new virus on Monday, bringing its total to 763 cases.

On Sunday, the country raised its disease alert to the highest level after a surge in infections and two more deaths.

South Korean President Moon Jae-in also ordered officials to take "unprecedented, powerful" steps to stem the spread of the outbreak.

Austria stops train from Italy due to suspected infections

Austria denied entry to a train from Italy on suspicion that two of the travellers might be infected with the coronavirus, Austria's Ministry of the Interior said.

"Tonight a train on its way from Venice to Munich was stopped at the Austrian border," the ministry said.

The Italian State Railways informed Austrian train operator OBB that there were two people with fever symptoms on the train, the ministry's statement said.

The train was now waiting at the Brenner Pass in Italian territory. "The further procedure is currently being discussed together with Italian authorities."

France, EU partners to discuss coronavirus: French health minister

French Health Minister Olivier Veran said he would talk to his European counterparts soon to discuss how to best cope with a possible epidemic risk in Europe as Italy battles an explosion in cases.

"Tonight there is no epidemic in France. But there is a problematic situation at the door, in Italy, that we are watching with great attention," Veran told a news conference.

"The situation tonight is very evolutive at [the] international level," he added. "I spoke with my Italian and German counterparts ... We have agreed to have a discussion between several European health ministers, probably next week, to assess how we can together face epidemic risk," he said.

A third person dies in Italy

A third person infected with the coronavirus died in Italy, a regional official said, as the government struggles to contain an outbreak of the illness in the north of the country with more than 130 cases reported since Friday.

Lombardy regional councillor Giulio Gallera told reporters the victim was an elderly woman from the province of Cremona in the Lombardy region.

THE CORONAVIRUS OUTBREAK IS A TEST FOR CHINA'S TECH INDUSTRY

China has spent decades nurturing its tech sector. Now, faced with a massive public health crisis, Beijing is pushing its tech companies to join the fight against the novel coronavirus. The country's tech giants have responded to the outbreak by deploying autonomous vehicles to bring supplies to medical workers, fitting drones with thermal cameras to improve detection of the virus and lending their computing power to help develop a vaccine.

It's not clear how much tech can help control the virus, which has now infected at least 79,000 people worldwide and killed more than 2,600, mostly in mainland China. And some of the efforts put forth so far are limited in size and scope.

But Beijing has made clear that fighting the virus is a national priority that requires collective action. The government has long stressed technological innovation as an important pillar of growth, and Beijing has spent billions of dollars on subsidies, loans and bonds designed to spur advancements in artificial intelligence, autonomous vehicles and other areas as it works to develop a tech sector that can compete with Silicon Valley.

"The fight against the epidemic cannot be achieved without the support of science and technology," Chinese President Xi Jinping said earlier this month, according to state news agency Xinhua.

He added that China should ramp up clinical research for vaccines and antiviral drugs, as well as expand online shopping options for the tens of millions of people who are staying indoors to prevent the disease's spread. The Chinese Ministry of Science and Technology on Thursday called on the tech sector for help, suggesting that robots, temperature screening machines and devices that can help reduce human contact should be deployed.

China's technological rise

China's efforts to create its own Silicon Valley date to the 1980s, when authorities began designating parts of the country as "high-tech development zones" focused on consumer electronics and biotech, among other fields. Those 168 zones reported more than 33 trillion yuan ($4.7 trillion) in revenue in 2018, according to official statistics.

Inside China's Silicon Valley: From copycats to innovation

Tech is also the linchpin of Beijing's "Made in China 2025" initiative, a plan to shift the economy from manufacturing to high-tech sectors. The mandate entailed investing billions of dollars of government funding into areas such as wireless communications, microchips and robotics. The focus on tech has worked. China was home to nine of the world's 20 most valuable tech companies in 2018 — a big leap over the two it claimed five years earlier, according to a report by venture capital firm Kleiner Perkins.

As China now fights the coronavirus, technology won't be the "dominating factor" that stops the outbreak, according to Danny Mu, a Beijing-based analyst of emerging technologies at Forrester. But he said the sector has its uses, including offering digital services like food delivery and mobile payments that help people "better face the epidemic."

Researching cures and eliminating human contact

This month, Tencent (TCEHY) opened up its super-computing facilities — which include machines that can run calculations much faster than an ordinary PC — to help researchers racing to find a cure. The Beijing Life Sciences Institute and Tsinghua University are among the participants.

And Didi, China's biggest ride-hailing provider, has teamed up with medical and aid organizations to allow workers who need to perform tasks related to data analysis, online simulation or logistical support to use Didi's servers for free.

Others are deploying robots to eliminate human-to-human contact. A robot operated by Meituan Dianping brings food to a customer at a restaurant in Beijing. "Yes, you can call them gimmicks," said Eliam Huang, an analyst at Coresight Research. "But Chinese tech companies can be very responsive and versatile." The food delivery giant Meituan Dianping, for example, introduced robots last week in some of its partners' restaurants in Beijing that help bring food from kitchens to delivery workers, and to customers waiting for takeout orders. Meituan wants to expand the program to other cities if it's successful.

Chinese e-commerce giant JD.com (JD), meanwhile, recently enlisted self-driving robots to bring goods to medical workers in the central Chinese city of Wuhan, where the virus originated. The bots, which look and run much like pint-sized vehicles, have been delivering packages to a hospital that primarily treats coronavirus patients. The route is relatively short — about 600 meters to the hospital — but cutting humans out of the equation has helped protect customers and employees, said Qi Kong, head of autonomous driving at JD Logistics.

An autonomous delivery robot making its first delivery to a hospital in Wuhan earlier this month. "As we learned of the situation in Wuhan, we started to pivot our resources there," Qi told CNN Business. "Time has been really tight. It only took us four days to make sure our algorithm was ready to go, from simulation to practice."

And a startup, Shanghai TMIRob, is sending dozens of robots inside hospitals throughout Wuhan, according to Chinese state media. There, they are spraying disinfectant in isolation wards, intensive care units and operating rooms.

Surveillance concerns

Drones have also been put to use during the outbreak. The technology allows authorities to scan through large crowds and spot if someone's in need of medical attention, according to MicroMultiCopter, a drone startup based in Shenzhen that has dispatched about 100 of the devices across the country. They've also sent nearly 200 employees to command centers where they can monitor what the drones are seeing in real time.

"The company has been working overtime," a spokesperson told CNN Business. "This is the best test of our drone system. It is also the best showcase to the world." The use of drones and other technology has opened up the country to criticisms about its vast surveillance state, which human rights groups have warned can be used to violate freedoms.

China has long used facial recognition, artificial intelligence and other technologies to crack down on crime and monitor its citizens. And tech companies like Tencent have for years been accused of censoring politically sensitive topics online in China. (The company has said before that it "respects and complies to local laws and regulations" of countries where it operates.)

China's tech sector has long benefited from "top-down" support from Beijing, said Huang, the Coresight Research analyst. The central government allocated 3.9% of the national budget to science and technology last year, a 14% increase over the year before. "This shows the government highly values the development of technology, and its dedication to push technology innovation forward," she said.

"Authorities' support helps everything happen faster," she added. "However, there is little ethical resistance, less ethical review in China."

3

The Impact of First and Second Wave of COVID-19 Pandemic on Global Society

The goal of this study is a comparative analysis of the first and second wave of the Coronavirus disease 2019 (COVID-19) to assess the impact on health of people for designing effective policy responses to constrain negative effects of future pandemic waves of COVID-19 and similar infectious diseases in society. The research here focuses on a case study of Italy, one of the first countries to experience a rapid increase in numbers of COVID-19 related infected individuals and deaths.

CORONAVIRUS SECOND WAVE

Human behavior is the major factor. State and local governments, as well as individual people, differ in their response to the pandemic. Some follow COVID-19 precautions, such as physical distancing, hand-washing and mask-wearing. Others are not as prescriptive in requiring these measures or in restricting certain high risk activities.

In some cities, towns and communities, public places are closed or practicing limitations (such as how many people are allowed inside at one time); others are operating normally. Some government and community leaders encourage or even mandate mask wearing and physical distancing in public areas. Others say it is a matter of personal choice.

However, the relationship between those precautions and cases of COVID-19 is clear: In areas where fewer people are wearing masks and more are gathering indoors to eat, drink, observe religious practices, celebrate and socialize, even with family, cases are on the rise.

Also, places where people live or work closely together (multigenerational households, long term care facilities, prisons and some types of businesses) have also tended to see more spread of the coronavirus. Coronavirus outbreaks at nursing homes and "superspreader" events — gatherings of people where one infected person or more transmits the virus to many others — continue to occur.

Are the spikes in coronavirus cases due to more coronavirus testing? No. During a surge, the actual number of people getting sick with the coronavirus is increasing. We know this because in addition to positive COVID-19 tests, the number of symptomatic people, hospitalizations and later, deaths, follows the same pattern.

COVID-19: Why are surges occurring across the U.S.?

Infectious disease expert Lisa Maragakis explains why COVID-19 cases are surging across the United States and important preventative steps to halt coronavirus transmission.

"Reopening" and Coronavirus Spikes

As communities began to reopen bars, restaurants and stores during the spring and summer of 2020, people were understandably eager to be able to go out and resume some of their regular activities.

But the number of people infected with the coronavirus was still high in many areas, and transmission of the virus was easily rekindled once people increased their activities and contact with each other. Medical experts urged reopening communities to continue diligent COVID-19 precautions, including physical distancing, hand-washing and mask-wearing, and monitoring for symptoms. Unfortunately, the combination of reopening and lapses in these infection prevention efforts has caused the number of coronavirus infections to rise again.

Tracking Coronavirus Surges

There is a delay between a policy change such as reopening businesses or relaxing occupancy limits in a community and when the effects of this change show up in the COVID-19 data. An increase in the number of COVID-19 cases or hospitalizations will not be seen a week or even two weeks later. It seems to take much longer, perhaps as many as six to eight weeks, for effects of a policy or widespread behavior change to appear in the population-level data.

When a person is exposed to the coronavirus, it can take up to two weeks before they become sick enough to go to the doctor, get tested and have their case counted in the data. It takes even more time for additional people to become ill after being exposed to that person, and so on. Several cycles of infection must occur before a noticeable increase shows in the data that public health officials use to track the pandemic.

So when an area relaxes precautions, the effects of that change will take a month or more to be seen. Of course, surges also depend on the behaviors of people when they start moving around more. If everyone continues to wear masks, wash their hands and practice social distancing, reopening will have a much lower impact on transmission of the virus than in communities where people do not continue these safety precautions on a widespread basis.

Is COVID-19 worse in the fall and winter? In the beginning of the pandemic, some people wondered: Will the coronavirus go away in the summer? Unfortunately, a substantial spike during the hot summer months in the U.S. made it clear that this was not the case. Other respiratory illnesses, like colds and influenza (flu), are more common in the colder months. Now that fall is here, we are seeing a dramatic increase in COVID-19 across the U.S. In colder months, people gather indoors and this is a risk for further transmission of the virus.

Why are experts concerned about future spikes of the coronavirus or a second wave in some areas? When the coronavirus first appeared in the U.S. in early 2020, it started with a very small number of infected people, so it took longer to spread. Now that the disease is widely distributed, with many unknowing coronavirus carriers in many different areas of the country, the risk of transmission is widespread.

Fall and winter in the Northern Hemisphere means inclement weather in many areas, with more people spending time indoors. Several holidays take place around the end of the calendar year, and people who celebrate them want to gather, travel, and visit friends and family.

Also, after many months of canceled activities, economic challenges and stress, people are frustrated and tired of taking coronavirus precautions. All these are factors that are driving surges and spikes in COVID-19 cases.

What is herd immunity from the coronavirus? Herd immunity is a public health term that refers to the fact that, when enough people in a community have immunity from a disease, the community is protected from outbreaks of that disease.

Infectious disease experts at The Johns Hopkins University explain that about 70% of the population needs to be immune to this coronavirus before herd immunity can work. People might be immune from the coronavirus, at least for a while, if they have already had it, but we don't know this yet. A widely available, safe and effective vaccine may not be available for months.

Without a vaccine, most doctors and scientists agree that a herd immunity approach of letting the virus "take its course" is not acceptable. Letting the coronavirus circulate freely among the public would result in hundreds of thousands of deaths and millions more people left with lasting lung, heart, brain or kidney damage.

Researchers are currently trying to determine if, and for how long, people are immune from the coronavirus after recovering from COVID-19. If it turns out that immunity only lasts for a while, people could get COVID-19 again, resulting in even more death and disability.

THE SECOND WAVE OF COVID-19 IN INDIA

Because an asymtomatic person, who carries the virus, would have spread the infection. In India, experts say, 80-85% of the population are asymptomatic. They continue to be the largest carrier of the virus, and in a closed indoor setting, asymptomatic person will transmit the virus even when he or she is talking. Also, asymptomatic people don't isolate themselves in a home setting.

A combination of a large asymptomatic population and the presence of more infectious variants of the virus during the second wave, which is much steeper than the first wave that peaked in September, continues to transmit the virus even to those who are staying indoors. For instance, the UK strain detected in a significant proportion during genome surveillance in Delhi and Punjab, has shown a 50% higher transmission, according to the US Centers for Disease Control and Prevention (CDC). The L452R mutation found in the variant B1.671, first detected in India, too has been associated with increased infectivity.

Second, in the current wave, the marking of containment zone has been less strict. In cities, the government has asked civil authorities to adopt micro-containment: with perhaps just a floor or a house defined as a containment zone. If there is no effective monitoring in micro-containment zones, containing the virus becomes a challenge. Earlier, an entire apartment or area would be made a containment zone, reducing the chances of transmission of the virus. Now, central teams have red-flagged the fact that high-risk contacts in workplace, social and family settings were not investigated and listed in Maharashtra, resulting in a surge. This is happening across the country.

Super-spreading events in indoor settings — house parties, social gatherings — can trigger local outbreaks if Covid-appropriate behaviours are not followed. Because some virus variants are more infectious, and because micro-containment zones are not being monitored as effectively as containment zones last year, we are seeing entire families going down with the virus. Contact tracing guidelines are not being followed as rigorously as last time. All asymptomatic direct and high-risk contacts of confirmed cases are to be tested once between day 5 and day 10 of coming into contact, but they can continue spreading the infection if they return a false negative result.

Also, during this surge, there has been a long waiting period for testing. Until the results are available, many asymptomatic persons violate isolation guidelines and spread the infection.

The infection is spreading at a faster pace in every age group. At present, there is very little data that shows how long immunity lasts in the younger population. However, those who have comorbidities at a young age at high risk.

Data released by the Centre shows that in seven age groups up to 70 years, the prevalence of deaths in this wave is comparable to the prevalence in the last wave. However, in the age groups 70-80 and above 80, mortality rates are higher in the second wave are higher. It is still the older population who is at higher risk and needs to be protected. However, the number of deaths are high in all age groups because there are more cases. And with the virus becoming more infectious and some mutations escaping the immune response, the younger population needs to strictly follow Covid-appropriate behaviours.

How did the medical oxygen situation turn this catastrophic? In the second wave, critical data has emerged from hospitals being tracked by the government — that 54.5% of admissions during the second wave required supplemental oxygen during treatment. This marked a 13.4-percentage-point increase from the peak during September and November last year, according to data from 40 centres across the country.

For moderate cases, India's clinical management protocol recommends oxygen therapy as the primary form of treatment: the target is to achieve 92-96% SpO2, or 88-92% in patients with COPD. It is this category that requires oxygen beds. While the proportion of those requiring oxygen beds is still hovering around under 10%, this number is at an all-time high with India's active caseload crossing 26 lakh.

As of April 24, official records showed that Delhi, UP, Gujarat and Haryana face severe shortfalls due to a surge in cases. The demand for medical oxygen has increased by 18% over the last six days across 12 states, which account for 83% of India's active cases.

SECOND WAVE OF COVID-19 SPREADING QUICKLY

The second wave of coronavirus infections has been spreading fast, which has caught even the medical officials by surprise. During the first wave, which was experienced last year, on an average 150 suspected cases would come for testing everyday. But this time the number of suspected cases who are coming for getting tested in Medak district alone has crossed 300 everyday, for the past few days. Officials are fearing that the number may soon rise exponentially.

"In the past, we used to get one or two cases from a family if a person tested positive for COVID-19. Now the situation is very different. Virus has been spreading through air. If one person in a family got infected with virus and there are 10 members in the family all the 10 are testing positive for the virus," said District Surveillance Officer Naveen. The variant strain (mutated virus) may also be another reason for fast spread of the virus, he added.

Dr. Naveen said that the number of deaths are also increasing to alarming levels. "During last year patients used to have a time of day or two to get admitted in the hospital. But this time round they do not have that luxury. Patient who appear normal are going out of control within an hour of developing dyspnea (medical term for shortness of breath) and death is taking place within no time. Many patients are asymptomatic and they do not know that they are carrying the virus. More than 70 % are asymptomatic," he explained.

Meanwhile the forest department officials held a massive vaccination drive in the district headquarters on Friday. "We have taken up this drive to clear all misgivings about vaccination among the staff. Similar programme will be organised for their families," said District Forest Officer G. Gnaneswar.

However, on Saturday vaccine shortage was reported at some places and it was confirmed by a medical officer in the Medical and Health department. At least one centre was reportedly closed due to lack of stock while at another centre the patients were given appointment for vaccination on Sunday. The stock was expected to reach Saturday night.

The streets of most places in the erstwhile undivided Medak district wore a deserted look due to fears among the people due to the surge in COVID-19 infections. The OP department of government hospitals were also shut down to minimize the spread of infection.

At some places in the town and the district residents were erecting barricades to prevent others entering their area.

NEW SYMPTOMS OF THE COVID-19 SECOND WAVE INFECTION

"Shortness of breath or difficulty in breathing (dyspnea), is one of the early symptoms of coronavirus, predominantly seen in infected patients during the

    Coronavirus & its Impact on the World Economy

second wave of COVID-19. Although the intensity of breathlessness can vary among individuals, this symptom leaves most patients with a feeling of tightness of the chest, resulting in the constant gasping of air, every few seconds," says Alexander.

Studies suggest that breathing difficulties are commonly seen in the second wave of COVID-19 patients, right at the onset of the infection. The infection causes a decrease in oxygen saturation (SO_2 levels) which may result in lung damage and in some cases, even multiple organ failure.

Besides this, other newer symptoms of the second wave of COVID-19 infection, that you must be aware of include :

1. Gastrointestinal tract infections: Your GI tract comprises the main organs of digestion, including the mouth, food pipe, stomach/gut, small and large intestine. Any disturbances in your GI system can wear down your immunity and hamper overall health. Symptoms of GI tract infections associated with COVID-19 include loss of hunger, vomiting, abdominal pain, and loose stools.

2. Hearing loss: Hearing loss is one of the symptoms in the second wave of COVID-19 infection. It may range from mild, moderate to severe which results in a sudden hearing loss, impaired hearing, or ringing sound in your ears (tinnitus). This starts early in the first week of infection and resolves over a period of time.

3. Extreme lethargy and weakness: Extreme weakness and lethargy have been reported as one of the early symptoms of the COVID-19 infection, more so during the second wave.

   Once your body identifies the COVID-19 virus (SARS-CoV-2) as an invader, it initiates the immune response to fight the virus, and this can result in the infected person feeling tired and weak.

4. Pink eye or conjunctivitis: Pink eye is an infection of the eye which results in the swelling of the outer transparent membrane (called the conjunctiva) of your eyelid and eyeball.

   Common symptoms include itching, redness, and tearing of the eyes, which results in puffy or watery eyes.

   Certain studies have explored the link between COVID-19 and ophthalmological (relating to the eye) symptoms. The COVID-19 virus is primarily transmitted through infected droplets in the air when someone sneezes, speaks or coughs. You can also pick the virus from infected surfaces and then touch your eyes, nose, or mouth, increasing the probability of infections of the eye, along with the nose and mouth.

   The new strains of the novel coronavirus in India are known to infect the conjunctiva. Unlike normal conjunctivitis, which usually affects both your eyes, conjunctivitis with COVID-19 is seen predominantly in one eye. It may be accompanied by constant eye irritation and sensitivity to light.

5. Dry mouth or not enough saliva: Saliva is the watery, frothy substance produced in your mouth that helps in digestion and keeps your teeth and mouth moist and healthy. When sufficient saliva is not produced by the concerned glands (salivary glands), it leads to a condition called dry mouth, which can lead to tooth and gum diseases and make you susceptible to infections. Dry mouth is now a common and initial symptom of COVID-19. Since the oral cavity (mouth) is a potential entry point for the novel coronavirus, it can attack the tissues and mucus lining your oral cavity, resulting in decreased saliva production and thus, dry mouth. Like the dry mouth, other oral manifestations of the coronavirus infection could be a dry tongue, changes in the colour and texture of your tongue, sores or blisters, and difficulty in eating.

6. Diarrhoea: Diarrhoea or loose watery stools is one of the widespread symptoms seen in COVID-19 patients during the second wave. Reports suggest most individuals affected with COVID-19 complained of persistent diarrhoea for 1 to 14 days, with an average duration of 5 days. Since diarrhoea is not usually thought to be a symptom of COVID-19 and can be a result of other digestive issues, there is a delay in getting tested for COVID-19 and hence, a delay in the identification of potential COVID-19 positive patients.

7. Headache: Sudden headaches can be a symptom of COVID-19. A normal headache that continues for a long time and does not subside with painkillers, is being reported as one of the newer symptoms seen during the second COVID-19 wave.

8. Skin rashes: Recent studies have highlighted skin rashes as a new symptom of COVID-19. Patients have reported rashes on their hands and feet, which are usually called acral rashes. Studies suggest that these rashes can develop as a result of the immunological response to the virus.

   If you develop any of the above symptoms, do not panic. It is advisable to isolate yourself from other family members and get yourself checked for COVID-19, after consulting your doctor.

   Additionally, if you have difficulty in breathing, tightness in the chest or chest pain, pale or blue-coloured skin, a sudden loss of speech or movement, or new confusion, seek medical care immediately.

9. Unexplained fatigue. Many people who tested positive for COVID-19 have reported feeling tired and fatigued prior to developing any other symptoms. In fact, in some cases, people don't have any other symptoms other than feeling fatugue and tired.

SECOND WAVE COVID-19 PANDEMICS IN EUROPE

A second wave pandemic constitutes an imminent threat to society, with an immense toll in terms of human lives and a devastating economic impact. The disease diffusion dynamics is traditionally modelled via compartmental1 or complex network diffusion techniques. These models provide a fairly accurate description of the time evolution of the number of affected individuals. However, it is a hurdle to predict the future evolution of a pandemic and to account for the diffusion across different regions of the World. Here we show that the epidemic Renormalisation Group framework is a simple and effective method to provide robust projections of the time evolution of a pandemic across regions. We apply it to the COVID-19, calibrating it on the first wave data, to efficiently simulate an incumbent second wave across Europe. We perform statistical analyses averaging on different levels of human interaction across Europe and with the rest of the world, finding that the second wave will occur between July 2020 and January 2021. Our results demonstrate that our method can be employed to describe pandemic dynamics beyond the European example. We anticipate that our results can be functional to a more quantitative understanding of future pandemics, which are expected to become a recurrent threat to our society. Our temporal playbook of the second wave pandemic can be used by governments, financial markets, the industries and individual citizens, to efficiently time, prepare and implement local and global measures.

Pandemics are increasingly becoming a constant menace to the human race, with COVID-19 being the latest example. A second wave is creeping back in Europe and is poised to rage across the continent by fall 2020. In this letter we provide a statistical analysis of the temporal evolution of the second wave of infected cases, with the impact for various European countries. To model the spreading, we employ the *epidemic Renormalisation Group* (eRG) framework. It can be mapped into a time-dependent compartmental model of the SIR type1. The Renormalisation Group approach has a long history in physics with impact from particle to condensed matter physics and beyond. Its application to epidemic dynamics is complementary to other approaches.

IMPACT ON INDIAN ECONOMY AFTER THE COVID-19 SECOND WAVE

It has been more than a year and a half since the COVID-19 pandemic penetrated the deepest core of human civilization and made us realize the power of mother nature. In India, after the first wave, we thought that we had gained control of the situation but the second wave found us wanting for basic necessities such as oxygen and medical supplies. It might appear that the second wave is on its way out with daily cases coming down to under 60,000 from the peaks of nearly 4 lakh cases, but we have lost over 3.8 lakh precious lives to COVID-19 already. With the hope that the situation will significantly improve on the medical side, it is time to assess the impact of the second wave on macroeconomics.

The government's approach in dealing with the two waves has been different. The response to the second wave has been localised and driven by the states while in the first wave we went for a national lockdown. I attribute this to the economic compulsions of the hard-hit central government and progressive spread of the virus. The second wave started in the west with Maharashtra, went up North and now is peaking in the south of the country. This spread journey makes a national lockdown economically suboptimal.

To understand the economic impact of the second wave, let's remind ourselves of the first wave and its impact on the economy. In the first wave, we went through a prolonged national lockdown and a significantly lower number of peak cases.

Manufacturing and the urban economy had come to a grinding halt while the rural economy continued to move because of less strict lockdowns. As a result, agriculture, which is the primary driver of our rural economy providing employment to 58% of our population, continued to grow.

Agriculture further benefited from good monsoon and cheaper and higher availability of labor. Reflecting on the GDP figures, our agricultural economy grew by 3.4% while the overall economy contracted with 7.7% in FY21. The first wave was primarily urban in its spread.

Urban areas reported more cases than rural areas for the first five months of the spread. In the second wave rural areas started reporting more cases than urban ones from the second month itself. An analysis of more than 50 most severely hit districts, 26 were in rural areas. Rural areas in the state of Maharashtra, Andhra Pradesh and Kerala were the worst impacted. The situation was further aggravated, due to the inadequacy of medical infrastructure in the rural areas and the rush of patients from villages and smaller towns to urban centers.

Agriculture

The second wave has seen stricter and longer lockdowns in the rural parts of the country. Due to the lockdowns, APMC Mandis have been closed for operations or have taken such steps voluntarily. Specifically, APMC Mandis in Gujarat, Rajasthan and Maharashtra were closed during the peak harvesting season. Farmers were not prepared for the ensuing chaos. As the Mandis have still not opened fully, crops are rotting in the fields. Due to the closure of Mandis, vegetable vendors, and processing industries have also been hit. We can see the contrasting impact of the first and the second wave in the agriculture wage growth data. The average wage growth for the agriculture sector for the period of November 2020 to March 2021 has reduced to 2.9 percent (2nd wave) from 8.5 percent in April to August 2020 (1st wave).

Manufacturing

Manufacturing was at the receiving end in both the first and the second wave. To control the coronavirus spread, most of the manufacturing sector had to work at a lesser capacity or shut down. Non-essentials manufacturing was hit for longer and with more severe restrictions. The fear of prolonged lockdowns led to migration back to villages. In addition, the global and local supply chains had also not fully normalized after the first wave. This has meant higher cost of procuring raw materials for both small and large industries. As per the IHS Markit India Manufacturing Purchasing Managers' Index (PMI) in May 2021, PMI slumped to 50.8 from 57.5 reported in February. It is at a ten-month low.

Services

The services sector in the last two decades has become the bedrock of the Indian economy contributing to more than half of the GDP. But, our services and knowledge-based industries have been built on the manufacturing industry premise of the 18th century i.e. proximity and discipline of workers to the factory is critical in getting good output. We apply the same philosophy for our software engineers and telecalling workforce.

With the internet revolution this premise has proven to be an unnecessary legacy of the past. Now the workforce can be decentralized and anyone can work from anywhere till the time there is 4G internet. I do believe that COVID will prove a positive disruption for the services sector in the long run.

The first wave required a steep learning curve for the organizations to develop infrastructure and processes for remote working. For the employees, first wave lockdowns were a new paradigm and it took them some time to adjust to work from home and be productive. Prolonged lockdown and unlocking phases during the first wave ensured that both the employer and employee got into a rhythm and the productivity started reaching pre-covid levels. The second wave disrupted this rhythm. But the impact of the second wave has been localized and centered around groups of people with typical disruptions costing 3-4 weeks of productivity. My assessment is that the services sector will be the least hit from wave 2 from an output standpoint.

The overall impact on GDP

On May 31, the Indian government released the data for GDP that during the financial year 2020-21, GDP contracted by 7.3 percent. It is the most severe contraction from the time India got its independence. The reasons behind this trajectory are obvious – lockdown leading to the closing of business units, increasing unemployment rate and a significant decline in domestic consumption.

For the current financial year, the Reserve Bank of India has anticipated growth of 10.5 percent. But the rating agencies across the globe have downgraded it due to the impact of the second wave of COVID-19. Moody's initially projected 13.7 percent of growth for FY 2021-22, but later lowered it to 9.3 percent. The same goes with S&P Global Rating. They have lowered the 11 percent growth to 9.8 percent in case of moderate impact of the second wave, but for a worst-case scenario, it would be 8.2 percent. The ideas around a third wave are not helping the situation at all.

To summarize on the macroeconomic numbers of GDP, I expect a less severe impact of the second wave due to less strict, localized lockdowns and practically a lesser number of days in reaching the peak number of infections. Agriculture will see a deeper cut from the second wave compared to the first wave where it grew. Our hopes of economic revival are pinned to us having an express vaccination drive, which takes away the fear of a third wave and a revival of consumer confidence and spending.

SECOND WAVE OF CORONAVIRUS INTENSIFIES ACROSS EUROPE

By mid to late May, Europe had tamed the first wave of the coronavirus, but not eradicated it. Had Europe opted to pursue elimination of the virus, a second wave could have been avoided. But, on the whole, governments let down their guard. And then, complacency kicked in. Restrictions were substantially eased over the summer and into early autumn. Subsequently, as the weather cooled in September, people returned indoors to bars, restaurants, offices, and homes where the virus could easily spread.

In the past 10 days, the European Union (E.U.) has overtaken the U.S. in terms of new coronavirus cases per capita. Europe's regional director of the World Health Organization (WHO), Hans Kluge, has said that there has been an exponential increase in daily cases across all of Europe, including the U.K. and non-E.U. countries, with the continent now reporting a 7-day average of more than 1,200 deaths a day.

While all of Europe is experiencing the effects of a second wave of coronavirus infections, there are major differences in impact and response across individual countries.

The figure below shows that Europe's coronavirus resurgence is being led by several countries that also headed the first wave, including Belgium, France, Italy, the Netherlands, and Spain. But, the second wave also includes several countries that had been spared for the most part during the initial March onslaught, such as Poland and the Czech Republic.

The level of confirmed infections is presently much higher than in March and April in many European countries. This is partly owing to more testing than during the first wave. But, the alarming rise in test positivity – now double-digit percentages in many European countries – suggests the intensity of the spread of the contagion is strengthening. Hospitalizations and intensive care unit occupancy are steadily increasing, with a number of jurisdictions - for example, the region in and near Liège in Belgium, and the metropolitan Rotterdam area in the Netherlands - already reporting healthcare system capacity issues.

Overall, Europe's second wave is worse in terms of daily new cases, but this hasn't (yet) translated into aggregate hospitalizations and deaths that exceed the numbers seen in the first wave, though in many countries numbers of hospitalized Covid-19 patients are already nearing 60% of the peak levels last March and April. The three growth curves – cases, hospitalizations, and deaths – exhibit distinct slopes, with hospitalizations less steep, and deaths somewhat flatter still. An important caveat is that death is a lagging indicator. Many who die from Covid-19 spend more than four weeks in hospital. So, it is premature to draw definite conclusions about the trajectory of the deaths curve. A fourth curve to keep an eye on is excess all-cause mortality. Across most of Europe excess deaths are rising again.

Notably, in the U.S. the observed pattern thus far is that the second peak (focused on the sunbelt states during the summer) and now ascending third wave (concentrated in the Midwest and Northern Plains) is hardest in areas previously less impacted; while across Europe the second wave seems to be affecting many of the same hard-hit areas that were struck during the first wave. There are a few conspicuous exceptions to the rule, including Italy's Southern provinces which had largely escaped Covid-19, and are now being hit hard as well.

As with the second apex that primarily impacted the sunbelt states in the U.S. over the summer, the discrepancy between curvature in the case and death curves can be traced to numerous factors. More testing may be at the top of the list, especially as it pertains to a younger demographic and those with mild or no symptoms. Indeed, the median age of those testing positive is at least 30 years lower than of people who contracted the virus in March. Older age is a critical risk factor that is positively correlated with a greater degree of severity of symptoms as well as death. Also, we may attribute fewer aggregate deaths during the second wave to the availability of number of comparatively effective treatments.

Since last week, European countries have re-introduced varying levels of restrictions, though so far most jurisdictions, with the exception of Ireland and the Czech Republic, are resisting the kinds of draconian lockdowns imposed in March. The impact of Europe's second wave of coronavirus infections is being felt differently across different countries. Accordingly, policy responses have differed.

The raft of measures taken by European governments includes limits on gatherings outside households, mask and physical distancing mandates, closing of non-essential businesses, bars, and restaurants, and even curfews in some locales.

Until now, the Czech Republic has implemented the most restrictive set of measures, which includes the closing of schools for at least three weeks. The Netherlands and Germany have imposed what they're calling a "partial lockdown" that comprises a shuttering of bars and restaurants (except takeout) but does not include schools. Other countries like the U.K. and Italy have tightened opening times of restaurants, imposed local partial lockdowns, set stricter limits on gatherings, and further expanded mask requirements. These measures are intended to stave off full lockdowns. It's unlikely these softer measures will preempt the need to impose harsher steps in the very near future.

4

Third Wave of COVID-19 Impacts Countries Around the Globe

Although some businesses have re-opened and restrictions have loosened in the United States and Europe, a third wave of infections is affecting countries around the globe, including ones where Partners In Health (PIH) works.

The most recent wave, which is when there is a surge in the number of cases over a period of time in a particular region, has been documented in Haiti, Lesotho, and Sierra Leone, among other countries. While there are many factors that contribute to waves, one currently is the emergence of virus variants, such as the highly contagious Delta variant identified in 92 countries, as of June 21. First detected in India in October 2020, the variant continues to spread.

PIH's approach to building strong health systems and responding to emergencies relies on the five S's: staff, stuff, space, systems, and social support. In Haiti, a lack of "stuff," namely vaccines, has had a significant impact on the country's 11.5 million residents. As of June 30, COVID-19 vaccines have yet to become publicly available in the Caribbean nation. Additionally, "space" has posed a challenge, as some hospitals have reached their limit on the number of COVID-19 patients they can accommodate. Within the the network of hospitals and clinics supported by Zanmi Lasante, PIH's sister organization in Haiti, there are 73 beds—33 of which were occupied, as of June 28— for COVID-19 patients at Hôpital Universitaire de Mirebalais and Hôpital Sainte-Thérèse in Hinche, which are the only two ZL-supported facilities providing direct care to patients with COVID-19.

Across Africa, COVID-19 cases are surging by 20% on a weekly basis and are quickly approaching numbers documented during the peak of the first wave in July

2020. In Lesotho, where an influx of people are crossing the border from neighboring South Africa—which has the highest number of COVID-19 cases on the continent, cases are rising and particularly affecting Leribe and Butha-Buthe districts, which are supported by the country's national health reform, and Maseru district, where the central office is based.

In response to the current wave, PIH Lesotho continues to supply oxygen to hospitals; provide logistical support to transport vaccines and health care providers throughout the country; run a mental health and staff wellness program to help health care workers cope with COVID-related stress; and get more rapid antigen test kits, in addition to the 10,000 they recently donated to Lesotho's Ministry of Health.

In Sierra Leone, COVID-19 cases are increasing and are at their highest since the beginning of the pandemic. There is a significant need to increase surveillance, prevention, and case management. As PIH Sierra Leone responds to the current wave, the team is focused on treating patients and providing social support, as they prepare for anticipated challenges, including oxygen and ICU bed shortages. Amid the third wave, new restrictions including a curfew, suspended religious ceremonies, and limited occupancy on social gatherings, were announced on July 1.

The number of COVID-19 cases, and the resulting death toll, will only continue to rise in countries unable to properly prevent the virus' spread, care for and support the sick, and conduct comprehensive vaccination campaigns. PIH continues to advocate for equitable global COVID-19 vaccination distribution, especially considering only 0.9% of people in low-income countries have received at least one dose of a COVID-19 vaccine compared to 45% of people in high-income countries.

THE COMING THIRD WAVE OF CORONAVIRUS

Long Bets is a philanthropic website built with funds from Amazon billionaire Jeff Bezos. Anyone can post a prediction and a challenge the winner donates the money to charity. Lord Rees, the prominent British astronomer, placed a bet in 2017 that "bioterror or bioerror will lead to one million casualties in a single event within a six-month period starting no later than December 31, 2020." His friend and Harvard psychologist Steven Pinker took up the wager and lost. All bets are off as the pandemic cuts widening fatal swathe in India because of no trials and many errors.

In a podcast, Niall Ferguson, the author of *The Ascent of Money: A Financial History of the World*, scoffed at projections by investment banks and governments of a V-shaped recovery sometime in 2021: "If you believe that, I'll sell you a bridge... because there's no way this is going to be a V-shaped recovery." The pandemic in India shows a bridge that will not be crossed anytime soon, thanks to government confusion, ignorance, lack of expertise, unscrupulous data fudging, slow vaccination drives and misplaced Vaccine Maitri.

Experts warn of an imminent third Covid-19 wave even before the nation has a chance to recover. Delhi Chief Minister Arvind Kejriwal has declared that the national capital is in the grip of a fourth wave. Experts in the US are debating the existence of a fourth wave. *The Washington Post* saw a rise in cases that equalled the crest of 2020. Every day, India is breaking the previous day's records. "We kept warning that the pandemic was not over but no one was listening," Rakesh Mishra, senior principal scientist and director of the Hyderabad-based Centre for Cellular and Molecular Biology told *National Geographic* last month.

What is a wave during a pandemic? It is the curve of any outbreak that reflects the rise and fall of the number of cases over a defined period. For example, the common cold crests in winter and drops in warm weather. A wave ends only when the virus has been contained and cases have fallen exponentially. A sustained rise in infections indicates a second wave, which is what has happened in India and is spreading to other countries. Research in the US and elsewhere shows that the common cold virus is usually active between December and March. Annual epidemics like influenza are accelerated by social factors like schools opening.

Two Oxford University scholars who studied respiratory disease epidemics in the past 150 years found that the peaks of the waves differ. For example, the 1889-92 influenza epidemic had three waves with different degrees of virulence. Like with the second Covid wave in India, the second stage of the 19th century outbreak was worse for young adults. This was the case during the influenza pandemic in 1918 and 2009, the former being compared to the current contagion. Epidemics have the maximum impact on a country's future; reports suggest that the third wave puts children at the risk of a higher rate of infection.

"Right now, we know that post the current wave the most vulnerable group would be the children. The adults are all being vaccinated on priority. We do not have the authorisation to vaccinate those under 18 years. This could pose a problem later," says Upasana Kamineni, founder of URLife, a wellness platform, and Vice Chairman CSR, Apollo Hospital.

Experts like Ferguson are predicting many more waves, though their magnitude is not certain.

Dr Sanjay Rai, Principal Investigator of Vaccine Safety and Efficacy Trial at AIIMS, Delhi, is also a professor at its Centre for Community Medicine and part of the development team of Covaxin. Rai told *The Leaflet*, a news website which has on its advisory board economist Kaushik Basu and Kalpana Kannabiran, Director,

Council for Social Development, Hyderabad, that it is difficult to predict the number of Covid-19 waves in India with the available scientific evidence. Like Ferguson, Rai is of the opinion that the human race will have to live with the virus for a long time to come.

"The Spanish Flu hit the world in three waves; it affected 2/3rd of the world's population before it disappeared. But does this mean coronavirus will disappear after the third wave? No, there is no guarantee. We may see a few more and distinct waves in the coming years. After that, the virus will run out of evolutionary options and settle down as a more benign, endemic pathogen," explains Gauri Chaudhari, healthcare industry expert and author of *The Perfect Pill.*

Why do these waves occur? The well-known reason for multiple waves is the mutation in the genetic code of the coronavirus. A slow vaccination pace gives it more time to mutate and find ways to evade or trick antibodies. This "accelerates the appearance of new variants as the continued spread of the virus allows it to get 'trained' to detect and bypass antibodies, since the immune system merely looks out for the original strain," Brazilian virologist Renato Santana told the media. Fitch Ratings has warned that this delay would cause more epidemic waves in the future; the only silver lining is its prediction that the economic damage of Wave Two will not be as severe as in the first.

Vaccinations in India dipped even as two-thirds of all districts reported a 20 percent climb in infection. "Scientists and public health experts believe that herd immunity is impossible because the virus is changing too quickly. New variants are spreading fast. We have to do mass vaccination as early as possible," says Dr Varsha Phadke, Dean, KJ Somaiya Hospital and Research Centre, Mumbai.

The Brazil variant is today considered its most dangerous form, which researchers confirm is a combination of 18 different mutations that includes Brazilian, British and South African variants. Deadlier and more infectious than the original coronavirus, this new scourge is a genetic combo of around two-dozen previously known mutations. "It is as if these variants were evolving," Santana reportedly said.

Three triple mutant viruses were found circulating in India last month. Of these, two were found in Maharashtra, Delhi, West Bengal and Chhattisgarh. Genome scientist Vinod Scaria in New Delhi had tweeted that one of the new mutants has specific genetic and immune escape variants and first appeared in West Bengal in October. But the government, flush with success over the first wave, did not act.

What makes variants lethal? Variants can override vaccines and unleash severe diseases, according to the US Centers for Disease Control and Prevention. They are fast movers. The D614G mutant can spread more rapidly than the original coronavirus by infecting human respiratory epithelial cells. Death is common after infection. Moreover, the mutant can resist monoclonal antibodies effectively. "For various mutant strains, a booster shot of the vaccines will be required to protect against variants, yet the protocols are not yet in place," says Phadke.

According to the Institute for Health Metrics and Evaluation (IHME), an independent global health research centre at the University of Washington, daily deaths in India will peak at 5,600 in mid-May. It has projected 665,000 Covid deaths by August 1, 2021. "Without drastic measures to decrease social mixing and increase effective face mask use, the situation currently looks quite grim in India," the briefing said. The institute estimates that universal mask coverage could prevent 70,000 deaths and that if the vaccination target for every Indian above 18 is met on schedule, another 85,600 lives would be saved by August 1. The Indian government is confident that the current wave will peak soon and the crisis is due to different states experiencing different peaks.

The Modi government had contained the first wave with a draconian lockdown. Then what happened? Cases came down. Morality rates receded. Economic activity was resumed in a phased manner. If it was not for complacency and self-congratulation, India would have indeed been a viswaguru.

Dr Antony Fauci, one of the world's foremost infectious diseases experts, has advised repeating the lockdown. The government is weighing its options.

Principal Scientific Advisor to the Prime Minister K Vijay Raghavan had warned earlier in the month that even after infection rates subside, a third wave is coming. "We can't predict the timing, but it seems inevitable. We must prepare ourselves and be ready for it," he told the press. But he is not clear on its timescale. "We should prepare for new waves," he cautioned.

Because of low testing capacity and an opaque data policy, medical experts put India's actual tally at five to 10 times the official number. Over 10 million cases have been added in over four months, though it took more than 10 months to reach 10 million in the first wave. At a Supreme Court hearing in the first week of May on oxygen distribution, Justice DY Chandrachud ordered, "We may enter stage three and if we prepare today we may be able to handle it. Whatever stocks procured needs to be sent to hospitals. It's not about allocating it to the state but also the logistics to see that it is distributed to hospitals."

The situation is so dire that *atmanirbhar* and anti-China rhetoric is in the bin; Indian companies have placed orders for more than 60,000 oxygen concentrators with Chinese medical equipment manufacturers to meet the shortage of medical oxygen in India. The Centre, however, refuses to accept any outside advice, especially from experts who are critical of its Corona effort. The Indian Medical Association (IMA) asked the Union health ministry to "wake up from slumber" and expressed shock that its suggestions are "put in to the dustbin" and that the government is making decisions without understanding ground realities.

Is India ready to meet a third wave?

Sadly not. According to an IIT-Kanpur study, Wave Three is projected to rear its head in October. Government incompetence, especially the tortoise pace of bureaucratic decision-making, has much to answer for the Covid-19 mess. Even as the vaccination drive falters, the Sputnik vaccine from Russia was stuck in the Central Drugs Laboratory where it was being tested for efficacy and other factors - 10 days after its arrival. Only about 9.2 percent of the Indian population have received the first dose at least. Daily vaccination targets are just about past the four-to-five million mark.

On April 5, India logged the highest number of jabs as 43,00,966 recipients got vaccinated. But on May 9, the rate plummeted by 84 percent. If the Wave Three has to be countered, 60 crore Indians in the 18+ population category must get 120 crore shots in five months, starting now. But shortage is plaguing many states. Glitches in booking slots on the CoWin platform have prevented aspirants aged above 45 from getting their jabs. Fortunately, states are evolving their own containment policy. Delhi, Odisha, Maharashtra, Uttar Pradesh, Karnataka, Telangana and Andhra Pradesh have decided to float global tenders to procure vaccines.

Though there is every need to be prepared for possible mutations in the future, genome sequencing of Covid-19 is hardly on track and almost petered out after Wave 2. People are casual about social distancing and wearing masks, be it at super-spreader events like the Hardwar Kumbh Mela or Friday prayers in Hyderabad. "The only way forward is to follow Covid-appropriate behaviour religiously and keep on vaccinating as fast as possible. Some more vaccines are expected in India in the next month or so which would address the vaccine shortage adequately," says Dr Namita Jaggi, Chairperson-Lab Services and Infection Control, and Chief-Education & Research, Artemis Hospitals, Gurugram. Since viruses mutate rapidly, vaccines have to be modified accordingly.

There are lessons to be learned in slow political will and red tape marring the dismal way India's second wave is being handled, thereby causing unimaginable agony to the population. To meet the third wave, the government will have to hugely ramp up the availability of oxygen. Despite receiving emergency medical aid from the US, UK and Europe and Oxygen Express deliveries, the country has reached nowhere near oxygen sufficiency levels. There is no centralised coordination of oxygen supply and distribution. Red tape hampers timely deliveries; marooned equipment at Customs depots was released only after the media broke the story. Foreign aid languished in airports because SOPs for distribution were delayed. Ventilators bought with PM Cares funds were found faulty in states such as Delhi, Rajasthan and Punjab. Media reports claim that hundreds of ventilators purchased using the same fund lie unused in states, including Madhya Pradesh, Uttar Pradesh, Maharashtra, Bihar.

India does not possess the capacity to store liquid oxygen at very low temperatures. Kept in cryogenic tankers, it is transported to distributors, who convert it into gas for filling cylinders. The number of cryogenic tankers in India is alarmingly low. Wave 2.0 is devastating rural India; the infection rate in Uttarakhand went up by 1,800 percent after the Kumbh. Madhya Pradesh's BJP government found that 99 percent of returning devotes tested positive. Health infrastructure in small towns and villages is moribund.

According to a research paper '*Covid-19: Challenges and its consequences for rural health care in India*' in *ScienceDirect*, "There is currently a shortfall in health facilities: 18 percent at the Sub-Centre level, 22 percent at the PHC (Primary Health Centres) level and 30 percent at the CHC (Community Health Centres) level (as of March 2018). Although the number of facilities has increased over the years, the workforce availability is substantially below the recommended levels as suggested by the WHO. Rural India has 3.2 government hospital beds per 10,000 people. Many states have a significantly lower number of rural beds than the national average."

In this bewildering scenario, unless India's rural healthcare and oxygen capacity and storage are ramped up massively, Wave Three will be more devastating to life, livelihoods and the economy. "The doctor-population ratio in India is 1:1,456 against the WHO recommendation of 1:1,000. There's a sheer shortage of healthcare support even after recruiting medical students from other streams, so the pressure is enormous. In fact, the frontline healthcare workers are the most at risk of infection. So, we have to do all we can to also protect them," demands Alok Sharma, CEO, Bengaluru-based Shycocan Corporation, manufacturer of a one-of-its-kind "virus attenuation" device called Shycocan.

The paucity of credible experts jeopardises discussion and the formulation of an effective future Covid-19 strategy, which takes into account the rural reality. "The reasons for the surge are many. How quickly the authorities, who are at the helm of affairs, learn lessons, accept the shortfalls and start taking steps to mitigate the effect of the next surge will make all the difference. We encountered challenges in managing the first wave due to systemic faults in our society, healthcare services, and governance," says Dr (Prof) Gautam Sen, Chairman & Founder, Healthspring, a leading primary healthcare solutions provider in India. The IMA has been calling for a planned, pre-announced lockdown to curb the virus spread. They say the lockdown will give medical infrastructure and medical staff crucial time to prepare for the coming wave.

What is keeping victory back? The government is playing coy on data. Policy formulation is impossible without it. Official numbers regarding infection and mortality are undercounted, due to low testing and image paranoia since seven states will go to the polls next year. In an open letter to Prime Minister Modi, 400 scientists sought wider access to the granular testing data collated by ICMR since the pandemic struck. "The ICMR database is inaccessible to anyone outside of the government and perhaps also to many within the government," the appeal stated. The Union health ministry has an aversion to sharing Covid data. Information is not dynamic and is restricted to once a day.

Regular press updates were discontinued. And the information available concerns only state-wise cases that are active and discharged, and about deaths on a given day. There is no data on the age-group or risk profile of Covid patients in ICU or on ventilators. The number of asymptomatic or pre-symptomatic patients is a secret. No findings on Covid deaths by age in different regions exist. The full serological data remains in ICMR's sole custody. Such censorship hampers the assessment of the viral spread and estimation of Covid-19's fatality rate which should be a priority for preparing for Wave Three.

Desperation marks the actions of a government that is on the back foot. Emergency clearance has been given to a DRDO-produced anti-Covid-19 drug. Dr Surya Kant, Professor and Head Department of Respiratory Medicine, King George Medical University, Lucknow, says, "We have revisited some of the old molecules and have found ivermectin, originally introduced as an antihelminthic, to be an effective, safe and affordable therapeutic option in Indian settings for prevention and treatment of Covid-19."

However, explains a World Bank official based in Delhi, "There is no medicine extant to cure a virus, you have to sit until it runs its course. Like with HIV, antiretroviral drugs can only contain the virus from replicating. SARS-Cov-2 is no different."

In any great crisis, superstition has a field day. During the Black Plague, people in England tied live cats and dogs under their clothes to ward off the disease. That was centuries ago, but India has not deviated from the path. The gentle cow finds itself in the middle of a raging controversy. The Covidiot is a product of the times.

Medical professionals are distressed about cow dung cures - in Gujarat, people are visiting cow shelters to gather dung and urine to smear on their bodies and later wash them away with buttermilk. Last week, media reported a Covid-19 hospital in Gujarat where patients would be exclusively treated with cow piss, ghee and other bovine products. A UP MLA not only prescribed cow piss as a Covid cure but also demonstrated how to drink it. US officials confiscated the bags of an Indian passenger which contained cow dung cakes.

A Union minister tried to solve the pandemic crisis by shouting the slogan 'Go Corona, Go!' The Union Health Ministry paid money to examine the efficacy of the Gayatri Mantra to curb the coronavirus. Research shows that superstitions have a healing role to play during a crisis, like a pandemic.

"Superstitions are normal and in some cases may help relieve stress in times of crisis, for instance during a global pandemic," Emily Balcetis, a social psychologist and associate professor of psychology at New York University, told AARP, a US–based interest group focusing on issues of people over the age of 50. "You can't stamp out Covid, but holding a rabbit's foot in your purse might feel like it brings some control," she says. "A magical trinket that keeps me safe—it's an illusory sense of control," is her opinion.

Her theory has found support in Jane Risen, a professor of behavioural science at the University of Chicago. "In these times when life feels more out of control, research suggests that those are the moments that people turn to magical thinking and superstitions more," she says.

BBC researchers did 1,447 fact checks on five Indian websites, where 58 percent of posts were mostly related to false cures, lockdown rumours and conspiracy theories about the origins of the virus. Some other posts said meat prevented infection, while chicken and eggs caused it. WHO labelled as false a video that attributed a prediction of '50,000 Covid-19 deaths by April 15' to the health body. More recently a fact check by a news website proved that the pictures and videos about corpses being flung in the river in Bihar were not all of Covid cases, because the cause of death could not be verified.

Sheer confusion over medicines has thrown health response into disarray. In spite of no medical evidence about remsedivir's efficacy, the clamour for it led to black marketing and imports. Dr Vijaya Raghavan and a few colleagues wrote to the government warning that 'irrational and nonscientific' plasma therapy has no validity to save lives. The fear of forced quarantine has forced many villagers to seek help from quacks. Many fake doctors have been caught operating from tin sheds, orchards and even a truck.

It seems that the spiraling death rate is perceived by many state administrators as a performance report. Pandemic politics has worsened the endemic confrontation between the Centre and Opposition states. On April 29, Delhi High Court asked the Centre why it was giving various states more oxygen than they had demanded.

Vaccine politics has got worse. Last month, the Centre released 350 lakh Covishield doses for distribution of which Maharashtra, one of the worst-hit states, got only 17.43 lakh doses while the BJP-ruled Uttar Pradesh (44.98 lakh), Madhya Pradesh (33.76 lakh), Karnataka (29.06 lakh) and Haryana (24 lakh) received more.

Vaccine wastage by states is another issue. Tamil Nadu, Haryana and Punjab have the highest wastage of the coronavirus jab. Kerala, West Bengal, Himachal Pradesh reported zero wastage.

"Unity is strength. The fight against the pandemic will have to be collaboratively fought by all the people of the democracy. Effective participation from all the people will ensure that the pandemic can be curtailed and will not overburden the healthcare system which is relentlessly working to ensure the safe well being of all the affected people," says Dr Nanditha, Consultant General Medicine, Apollo TeleHealth, Hyderabad.

The government needs to adopt a transparent and non-partisan approach in treating Covid-19 to contain Wave Three and beyond. Honest data collation and exchange, accelerating vaccination, equitable distribution of aid, setting up more Covid facilities with beds, oxygen supplies and staff and expanding and empowering rural infrastructure will go a long way in meeting the challenge. Or else the pyres will keep burning late into the night of another year, or perhaps more.

Mumbai Shows the Way

Last week, the Supreme Court recommended the Mumbai Model to the Centre to manage oxygen supplies. The lessons learned during the first wave were applied by the Brihanmumbai Municipal Corporation (BMC) to prepare for the second. There are 31,695 Covid-19 beds, including 12,754 oxygen beds and 2,929 ICU ones, in the city.

The BMC conducted a survey of oxygen demand to identify vulnerable areas and entered into agreements with nearby private plants to procure liquid oxygen daily. Protocols were evolved to prevent oxygen waste. Experts trained medical professionals to achieve minimum consumption by monitoring saturation and leakage. Hence, 275 metric tonnes of oxygen were enough to satisfy the requirement of Mumbai's 90,000-odd active patients.

During the first wave, the BMC stopped refilling cylinders and opted for jumbo liquid medical oxygen tanks that can store 13,000 kilo litres, a 10-fold increase in capacity. Two of these cylinders each were installed in large hospitals to provide three to four days of oxygen supply. BMC has in reserve old cylinders which can supply patients for one to two days in case demand rises.

Cities like Bengaluru are taking cues from Mumbai. The Karnataka government has asked the Bengaluru city corporation to set up Ward Decentralised Triage and Emergency Response (Ward DETER) committees to ensure emergency medical care to critical Covid patients. A list of available hospital beds and oxygen resources will be updated in real time.

AFRICA FACING 'BRUTAL' THIRD WAVE OF PANDEMIC AS VACCINATION SLOWS

The Delta variant of the coronavirus, first detected in India, has so far been reported in 14 African countries, according to the World Health Organisation.

Africa is facing a vicious coronavirus resurgence, with unprecedented hospital admissions and fatalities pushing health facilities to the brink as the continent falls far behind in the global vaccination drive.

With just under 5.3 million reported cases and around 139,000 deaths among its nearly 1.3 billion people, Africa is still the world's least-affected continent after Oceania, according to an *AFP* tally.

So far, African nations have been spared disasters comparable to Brazil or India. But the pandemic is resurging at an alarming rate in at least 12 countries, with continental cases expected to hit a record peak in around three weeks.

"The third wave is picking up speed, spreading faster, hitting harder," World Health Organization Africa director Matshidiso Moeti warned Thursday. "The latest surge threatens to be Africa's worst yet". Africa Centres for Disease Control and Prevention (Africa CDC) director John Nkengasong on Thursday described the third wave as "extremely brutal" and "very devastating".

And Liberia's President George Weah has warned the wave is "far more alarming than a year ago" as hospitals overflow in his country. Compounding Africa's third wave are immunisation hitches, the spread of more transmissible virus variants and winter temperatures in the Southern Hemisphere.

The Delta variant, first detected in India, has so far been reported in 14 African countries, making up the bulk of new cases in the Democratic Republic of Congo and Uganda, according to the WHO. Doctors in South Africa, which accounts for more than 35 per cent of all cases recorded on the continent, are struggling with an unprecedented influx of patients.

Unlike past waves, this time "the hospital system is not coping," said doctors' association chief Angelique Coetzee. South Africa's average new daily infections have increased 15-fold since early April, with hospital admissions rising around 60 per cent.

'Unprecedented' Deaths In Zambia

Namibia and Zambia are also seeing steep infection curves. Zambia's health ministry has reported an "unprecedented" number of COVID-19 deaths piling pressure on mortuaries while Africa CDC said the country was "overwhelmed".

With similar trends in Uganda, Health Minister Jane Ruth Acheng blamed highly infectious variants for the new spread, "different from the second wave" with a large number of young people hospitalised. Uganda is one of the countries facing reported oxygen shortages, although Acheng denied civil society groups' claim that the shortfall amounts to 24.5 million litres per day.

Governments are again tightening restrictions, including a new nationwide lockdown in Uganda and a tougher curfew in 13 Kenyan counties. At the same time, the pace of vaccinations is struggling to get off the ground.

According to the WHO, about one per cent of the continent's population is fully vaccinated — the lowest ratio globally — and 90 per cent of African nations will miss a target to inoculate a tenth of their populations by September. "We are running a race behind time, the pandemic is ahead of us. We are not winning in Africa this battle against the virus," said Africa CDC's Nkengasong. "It's frightening what is going on on the continent," he added.

A recent pledge by Western leaders to donate one billion vaccine doses to poorer countries has been widely criticised for being too slow. Cases are "outpacing vaccinations", Moeti said. "Africa urgently needs a million more vaccines. We need a sprint".

'Waiting To Die'

Several countries have failed to administer jabs from the UN-backed Covax scheme before their use-by date because of logistical failures and vaccine hesitancy. Malawi destroyed almost 20,000 expired AstraZeneca doses in May, while the DRC and South Sudan have returned more than two million shots to the UN to avoid a similar scenario.

Authorities in Congo-Brazzaville are concerned over the slow take-up of almost 100,000 Chinese-made vaccines expiring in July. A surge in coronavirus cases in India, the world's main AstraZeneca supplier, has delayed Covax deliveries to Africa. Malawi exhausted its stocks last week, just as thousands were due for their second shot.

And hundreds of frustrated Zimbabweans protested last month after Harare's main vaccination centre ran out of jabs.

South Africa says it has secured enough Johnson & Johnson and Pfizer/BioNTech vaccines to immunise 67 per cent of its 59 million inhabitants. But the rollout has been hit by setbacks and only 2.2 million people — healthcare workers and over 60s — have received a jab so far. "The lack of vaccines in a region with high levels of poverty and inequality means many people feel they are just waiting to die," said Amnesty International's regional director Deprose Muchena.

FROM GERMANY TO CANADA, HOW COUNTRIES ARE COUNTERING A NEW COVID-19 WAVE

Several countries are extending or reintroducing lockdowns and restrictions as a third wave of the novel coronavirus sweeps the world.

The surge is fuelled by the new variants of the virus such as the B117 mutation first detected in the United Kingdom. It is said to be 50% more transmissible than the original virus and may also be more deadly. "The spread of the variants is driving the increase. But so is the opening of society when it is not done in a safe and a controlled manner," Hans Kluge, the WHO's Europe director, said.

Germany

After reopening schools in late February and allowing hairdressers and some shops to resume business in March, Germany may prolong its partial lockdown which ends on April 18 as the country recorded 29,000 new cases on Thursday. Most of those being infected were in the 15 to 49 age group, much younger than those in the first two waves.

The number of cases in the over-90s is also on the rise. Death rates have levelled off over the past two or three weeks, but not gone down. Almost 80,000 people in Germany have died of the virus.

Almost 5,000 ICU beds are taken up by Covid-19 patients, and the figure is expected to rise to 6,000 by the end of the month. Covid patients also made up 80% of those in hospital on heart and lung replacement machines to keep them alive, figures released by the Robert Koch Institute stated.

France

France entered its third national lockdown in early April to tackle a surge in cases of Covid-19 that threatens to overwhelm the country's hospitals. All schools and non-essential shops have been shut till the end of April and a curfew has been imposed from 7 pm to 6 am.

The country on Thursday became the latest one to record more than 100,000 deaths due to Covid-19. The threshold was reached after 300 fatalities were registered over the past 24 hours, bringing the official toll to 100,077.

Like other countries, Emmanuel Macron's government is also counting on vaccines to help bring the outbreak under control. By April 14, France had administered a total of 15.75 million vaccine doses, of which 11.6 million were first doses, according to data disclosed by health authorities.

Italy

New daily cases in Italy have surged from a weekly average of just over 12,000 in January to more than 20,000 in March and April with the country recording 16,160 new cases in the last 24 hours. According to the World Health Organisation, Italy has recorded 3,809,193 confirmed cases of Covid-19 with 115,557 deaths between January 3, 2020, and April 15, 2021.

More than half the country — including Milan and Rome — is already under the new regime, which placed any region with more than 250 cases per 100,000 automatically in the "red" category, meaning bars, restaurants and schools must close.

Netherlands

The Dutch government said on Thursday that early easing of lockdown will not be feasible as night-time curfew and other restrictions would remain until at least April 28 due to a rise in cases. This comes at a time when the country reported 5,503 cases on Wednesday, an almost 35% increase when compared to daily infections being reported a month back.

Earlier the government had said they were looking at easing restrictions on April 21 by lifting the curfew and allowing bars and restaurants to welcome guests in outdoor spaces.

Poland

The Polish government has extended the nationwide Covid-19 lockdown till April 25, saying the recent spike in cases have taken a toll on the country's healthcare system. On Wednesday, 21,283 people had tested positive in Poland. The country has so far reported 2,621,116 confirmed cases, while the death toll stands at 59,930.

The restrictions include one customer per 20 square meter in shops and places of worship while furniture and hardware stores larger than 2,000 square meters will stay closed. Hotels and other establishments offering sleeping facilities will have restrictions imposed till May 3.

Canada

Prime Minister Justin Trudeau has warned that Canada is fighting against a "very serious third wave of infections" as the new variant of the virus is spreading fast across the country.

"Around the world, countries are facing a very serious third wave of this pandemic," Trudeau told a press conference. "And right now, so is Canada."

Canada has averaged nearly 5,200 new coronavirus cases per day over the past week, and has recorded a total of more than a million positive tests and 23,000 deaths.

HAS COVID-19 FATIGUE CAUSED A THIRD WAVE IN EUROPE?

In early March, the WHO warned that the number of COVID-19 cases being reported across the continent of Europe was on the rise. Hans Kluge, Europe director at the WHO, urged leaders to "get back to basics" and re-engage their populations in the drive to contain the pandemic.

"Pandemic fatigue," he said, might be causing people to start to ignore social distancing measures, particularly combined with ongoing vaccination efforts which may also be encouraging people to relax a bit too much.

AstraZeneca COVID vaccine 76% effective in new US trial analysisWill rich countries lift waivers on patents for COVID vaccines?Greed is the problem, not the solution, for vaccine woesIs there a link between the AstraZeneca vaccine and blood clots?

It is in Central Europe, the Balkans and the Baltic states where case incidence, hospitalisations and deaths are now among the highest in the world. Furthermore, the WHO says, the number of people dying from COVID-19 in Europe – 20,000 a week – is now higher than it was this time last year.

In response to this, many European countries have re-introduced or extended lockdown measures. Germany has extended its current restrictions until April 18 and initially planned a five-day nationwide lockdown for the first five days of April but, after much backlash, Chancellor Angela Merkel reversed this decision.

Paris is entering a new month-long lockdown, together with several other regions in the north and the south of France. A total of approximately 21 million people in 16 areas of France will be affected. France already has a nationwide curfew from 7pm to 6am.

Shops, schools and restaurants are closed in many major Italian cities, including Rome and Milan. Italy has also planned a nationwide shutdown over the three-day Easter weekend, starting on Good Friday, April 2.

Although Greece has stated it is planning to welcome foreign tourists during the European summer, it, too, has introduced new restrictions in areas where cases are highest, including Athens where non-essential shops and hairdressers are closed.

Spain's current restrictions are in place until May and only essential trips out of the home are allowed.

All of these measures will come as a blow to Europe's pandemic-weary populations, who have seen themselves in and out of restrictions for a year now.

Many of these are the same countries that were successful at controlling the disease in the first six months of 2020, so where did it go wrong and what can be done to prevent it from getting worse?

The new variants have played a part. Some 48 out of 53 European countries or territories have reported the B.1.1.7 variant (PDF), first identified in the UK. It is known to be up to 50 percent more transmissible than the original variant of the coronavirus due to a mutation affecting its spike protein.

This mutation allows the spike protein to latch onto human cells more readily and with stronger bonds than the original, making it more likely to infect human cells and eventually become the dominant strain, more adept at thwarting measures that were previously effective.

Several countries where this variant has become dominant have seen rapid increases in the numbers of cases, resulting in increased hospitalisations, overstretched health systems and excess mortality.

Particularly badly hit is the Lombardy region of northern Italy, which includes Milan and saw very high numbers of cases in the first wave of the pandemic this time last year. Intensive care units there are, once again, filling up with patients, two-thirds of whom are thought to have been infected by the UK variant.

Also of concern is the B.1.351 – or South African – variant, which contains the E484k mutation, which can make it less susceptible to antibodies produced by a vaccine or by having previously caught COVID-19. This variant has been identified in smaller numbers in several European countries, including Spain, Germany, France and Italy, and is being carefully monitored by local governments.

Alongside all this is the worryingly slow rollout of vaccines across European Union member states. The EU ordered 300 million doses of the Pfizer-BioNTech vaccine but delivery has been delayed because the plant where the vaccine is made has undergone refurbishment in order to increase production in the longer term.

The supply of the Oxford-AstraZeneca vaccine to the EU has been a contentious issue. Oxford-AstraZeneca said it had supply chain issues at its plants in Belgium and the Netherlands, while the EU feels the UK has been prioritised for vaccine deliveries, even though it signed its contract with AstraZeneca later than the UK did.

In January 2021, despite the European Medicines Agency deeming it safe and effective for all age groups, several European countries including France, Belgium, Germany and Sweden decided the Oxford-AstraZeneca vaccine should not be used for people over the age of 65. This caused widespread damage to public confidence in the vaccine and slowed the rollout further. A month later, Germany, Belgium and Sweden reversed their decision, stating the vaccine was indeed effective in all age groups and France approved it for those aged 65 to 74. But at a time when vaccine scepticism is high, there is no doubt in my mind that this would have put some people off having the Oxford-AstraZeneca vaccine.

On top of this, there was the much-publicised halting of the Oxford-AstraZeneca vaccine in many European countries in March, about concerns it might be linked to the occurrence of blood clots. These claims were later dismissed by the European Medicines Agency, which, after reviewing the data, found no link between blood clots and the Oxford-AstraZeneca vaccine.

These small, but important, delays to the rollout of that vaccine have given the virus the opportunity to spread. The new lockdown measures being introduced by governments are designed to suppress this spread and reduce the risk of new variants emerging. Identifying and isolating breakouts of variants of concern will be key while the vaccine rollout is ramped up.

Foreign travel, so important to many European economies during the lucrative summer months, may well have to be restricted for another year. More difficult to manage will be the issue of "pandemic fatigue" in many of these countries where citizens' liberties have already been restricted for some time.

Expectations around the easing of lockdown measures will need to be carefully managed, a task that is easier said than done. Decisive and firm government measures may still yet stop this potential third wave from reaching the peaks of previous waves, but the time to act is now.

Towards the end of last year, a new COVID variant was identified in the blood samples of infected people in the US city of New York. Since then, we now know, it has spread at an alarming rate through the city.

The new variant, known as the B.1.526 variant is now thought to account for almost half of new cases in the city. A study has shown this variant has a number of mutations that distinguishes it from others, but two are of particular note: First

is the E484K mutation, also found in the South African and Brazil variants. This mutation changes parts of the spike protein of the virus to a degree where the immune response triggered by vaccines is not as effective. The second is the S477N mutation, which affects the part of the spike protein that binds to human cells, making it more effective. We do not know yet if this will make the virus more transmissible, but studies are continuing.

It is difficult to know how worried we should about new variants that keep cropping up. The studies into the New York variant are yet to be peer-reviewed and formally published, so it is worth taking a step back from the headlines and sticking to what we know works: Social distancing, hand washing and mask-wearing. For now, stick to the local guidelines and go for your vaccine when called.

In the Vaccine Clinic: Explaining to my patients why they must still wear masks Attending the COVID vaccine clinic is one of the best parts of my job. It sounds strange but, as a doctor, it is rare for me to finish a general clinic where everyone has been in a good mood. Covering a clinic will usually involve delivering bad news to a patient or finding something when examining someone that warrants further investigation. But at the COVID vaccine clinic, the clinical staff, the volunteers and the patients are all smiling, although it can be tricky to see behind our masks.

The vaccines have been billed as injections of hope; the way out of the pandemic. Because the vaccines are being given first to those at the highest risk of serious illness from COVID-19, it is mostly the elderly or those with underlying health conditions that we have been seeing.

These are the same people who have been told that they must stay indoors for the very reason that they are most at risk. These are the same people who had the most to lose if they catch COVID-19. In a year where many have not been able to see or hug their family members, it is only natural for them to want to know whether having the vaccine means they can ease up on social distancing measures.

Sadly the answer, for now, is no. The vaccines will help protect those vaccinated from serious disease or death if they do catch COVID-19, but we do not yet have definitive evidence that they reduce transmission.

Although preliminary research from Israel does suggest that transmission rates have come down following vaccination, this has yet to be concluded. Vaccination rates vary depending on which country you live in, but no country has yet vaccinated enough people to assume herd immunity – the threshold at which enough people are deemed sufficiently protected to ease lockdown measures. By wearing masks and socially distancing, you are protecting those who have yet to be vaccinated from contracting the disease.

Many people have asked me what the point of the vaccine programme is if not to remove lockdown and social distancing measures. That is indeed the long-term goal and global vaccination will play a huge part in that. But, today, the point of the vaccines is to stop people from getting sick from COVID-19 and potentially dying from this terrible disease.

For many people, repeated lockdown measures have had a devastating effect on livelihoods and mental health, and I understand that. But this pandemic is not yet over and, until it is, we must continue to adhere to local social distancing guidelines, even after having a vaccine.

5

Coronavirus: A Visual Guide to the Outbreak

The respiratory infection, which has been given the official name Covid-19, has claimed more than 2,000 lives so far - more than the 774 killed in the 2003 Sars epidemic. The outbreak, originating in the Chinese city of Wuhan, has been declared a global emergency by the World Health Organization (WHO). Here are 10 maps and graphics that will help you understand what is going on.

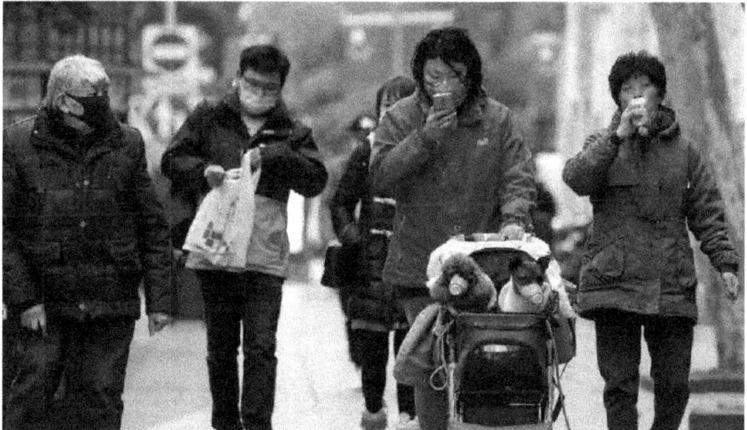

A fast-moving virus known as the "new coronavirus" has infected thousands of Chinese citizens and spread to more than 25 countries.

There have been thousands of cases - the majority in China

Across China, tens of thousands of people have been infected with the coronavirus, which causes pneumonia-like symptoms. Thousands more are under medical observation. Changes to the way patients were diagnosed briefly caused a spike in the figures, with a huge increase in the number of confirmed cases on 13 February.

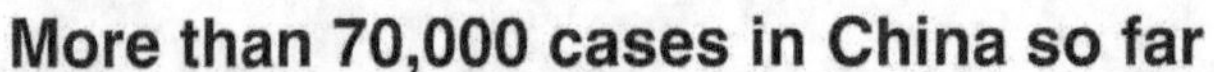

More than 70,000 cases in China so far

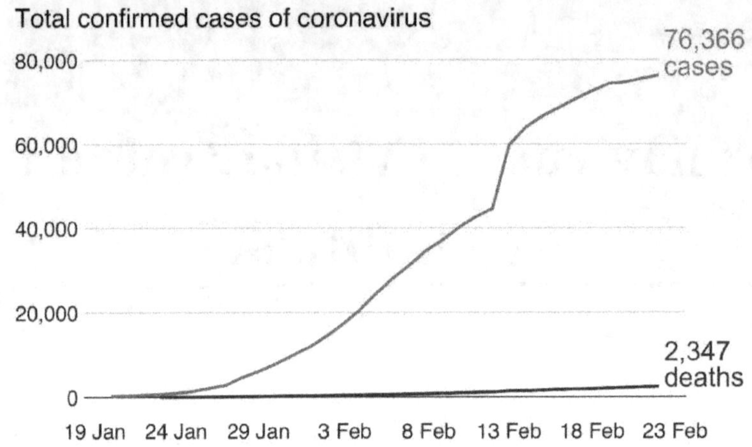

The change allowed doctors in Hubei province - the centre of the outbreak - to diagnose Covid-19 and begin treatment before receiving a positive test result for the virus, as long as a medical assessment and a chest scan suggested the patient might be infected. This change was later reversed, causing a dip in the number of cases recorded on 20 February.

On both occasions the province's health authorities confirmed they had revised existing data. This suggests many of the cases that caused the spike on 13 February were old cases being re-classified as coronavirus infections rather than new patients.

A study of 44,000 cases by the Chinese Centre for Disease Control and Prevention found that more than 80% had been mild, with the sick and elderly most at risk, while 4.7% had been critical. According to Chinese officials more than 18,500 people have recovered from the virus.

A VISUAL GUIDE TO THE WUHAN CORONAVIRUS

An outbreak of new coronavirus has sickened about 1,400 people worldwide and killed at least 41 in mainland China, while spreading to countries around the world. Its emergence has fueled fears of a deadly epidemic as hundreds of millions of people travel in China, or around the Asian region, during the Lunar New Year holiday.

What is the virus? Coronavirus is a large family of viruses, which include severe acute respiratory syndrome (SARS) and Middle East respiratory syndrome (MERS). Common symptoms include a runny nose, cough, sore throat, and possibly a headache. Those who have a weakened immune system, particularly the young and the elderly, are at risk of the virus turning into a more serious respiratory tract illness.

Authorities said the Wuhan coronavirus was passed from animals to humans; can be spread from person to person; and appears to cause pneumonia in people who have weakened immune systems. It is thought to be milder that SARS and MERS and take longer to develop symptoms. Patients to date have typically experienced a mild cough for a week followed by shortness of breath, causing them to visit a hospital.

Experts are now trying to understand how it is being transmitted, who is at most risk and whether transmission is occurring mostly in hospitals or in the community. In one instance, 14 doctors and nurses operating on a patient — who was not known to be carrying the virus — were all infected with it, suggesting it can be spread relatively easily. Where it started: Ground zero: The outbreak emerged last month in the largest city in central China, Wuhan, a city of 11 million people in Hubei province.

Officials linked it to Huanan Seafood Wholesale Market, saying wild animals sold there are the likely source of the virus. The market has been closed since January 1 for disinfection and officials are scrambling to discover its animal source.

Snakes — the Chinese krait and the Chinese cobra — may be responsible for transmitting coronavirus to humans. Scientists in China say that the virus might have jumped from bats to snakes, which were sold in the local seafood market in Wuhan, and then to humans.

However, how the virus could adapt to both the cold-blooded and warm-blooded hosts remains a mystery, and further tests are necessary to determine the source animal. At least 30 people died in the province, many of them elderly and suffering from pre-existing conditions. As deaths mount in the city, officials imposed a number of new measures including the postponement of New Year celebrations in Wuhan, a ban on tour agencies from bringing groups of people out of the city and thermal monitors and screening in public spaces.

Regional spread

From the first reported case in December, in Hubei province, the virus has spread to almost all of China's administrative regions this week. The country has adopted prevention and control measures that are typically used for major outbreaks such as plague and cholera. This means health officials will get sweeping powers to lock down affected areas and quarantine patients.

Wuhan "temporarily" closed its airport and railway stations on Thursday for departing passengers, and all public transport services are suspended until further notice. The city's coronavirus task force also announced the closure of highways out of the city. Meanwhile, the city made it mandatory for everyone to wear face masks in public places after confirmed coronavirus cases passed the 500 mark.

Unprecedented lockdown

Authorities in China have imposed indefinite travel restrictions in 15 cities in Hubei province, the most affected area in the country, impacting an estimated 32 million people. Wuhan, a city of 11 million, is under effective lockdown, with all public transport in and out of the city closed. Other cities across the province are under less severe travel restrictions.

A global threat: Confirmed cases around the world

The virus has spread well beyond mainland China, so far to 13 places including Hong Kong, Macau, Taiwan, Singapore, South Korea, Thailand, Japan, Vietnam, Australia and the United States. Airports around the world have increased health screenings and implemented new quarantine procedures as officials race to slow the spread of the virus. Various countries, including the US and the UK, have also issued travel advisories for Wuhan.

International flights from Wuhan

Wuhan is a major transportation hub. Not only is the city a center for China's high-speed rail network, it has flights going to more than 60 international destinations from Tianhe International Airport.

On Thursday, as confirmed cases ramped up across the country, government officials announced the temporary closure of Wuhan's airport and railway stations. All train tickets in and out of Wuhan have also been suspended, while multiple international airlines have canceled flights to the city.

China has encouraged passengers traveling to and from Wuhan to change their travel plans during the busy Lunar New Year holiday period, by exempting them from service charges for refunds for all modes of transport. How does this compare to the SARS virus? Scientists say the infectiousness of the virus is not as strong as SARS, but have added that the number of people infected is climbing.

A study by researchers in the UK estimated that the number of infections in Wuhan is still grossly underestimated, with the real number closer to 4,000 as of

January 18, based on the spread of the virus to other cities and countries in a relatively short period of time. SARS infected more than 8,000 people and killed 774 in a pandemic that ripped through Asia in 2002 and 2003.

On Thursday, David Heymann, the chairman of a World Health Organization committee gathering data on the outbreak, said the virus spreads more easily from person to person than previously thought. But there is still much that is not known about the virus and, as the above graphic shows, its death rate is far smaller than that seen during the SARS outbreak.

MISPLACED ANGER

People's concerns and anxiety about the coronavirus outbreak are understandable but that cannot be an excuse to malign the WHO or its chief. In times of an epidemic of this magnitude, people, irrespective of national boundaries and political leanings, need to stand united and support individuals and organisations that are working on ground to tackle the crisis. Hurling personal attacks on individuals leading such efforts doesn't help improve the situation, but rather often proves to be counterproductive. It infuses negativity in public discourse, which in turn tends to cast aspersions on genuine efforts—a breeding ground for suspicion and misinformation.

A confrontational approach against President Xi Jinping is likely to snowball and prove futile when it comes to controlling the situation. Secondly, one may have a hundred differences with China and what its political system and leadership stands for. But is this really the time to attack and malign the nation?

Before attacking Dr Ghebreyesus for meeting President Xi Jinping and praising his government's efforts against coronavirus, one must realise that besides leading an international health organisation in the midst of an epidemic, Dr Ghebreyesus also has to negotiate various diplomatic hurdles in forging an international coalition against the epidemic. With regards to coronavirus, this global effort is simply impossible if China is not on board.

Faced with such a sensitive situation, the WHO chief cannot afford to upset the Chinese leadership, even if there are some shortcomings on ground. A confrontational approach against President Xi Jinping is likely to snowball and prove futile when it comes to controlling the situation.

Those who are calling Dr Ghebreyesus names and demanding his resignation must answer if they think China would have allowed a WHO team comprising international health experts to visit coronavirus-hit regions and investigate the situation had the health body's chief confronted President Xi and talked bitter about him.

The reality today is that thousands of people are suffering in China. Many have died and many more are likely to die in the coming days. Priority for the global community right now should be to control the situation, not to embroil itself in mudslinging and waste its energy by pointing fingers in a show of one-upmanship. Investigations into who and what went wrong (if at all) can wait. Saving lives can't.

Dr Ghebreyesus's success in convincing China to allow a team of international health experts to visit coronavirus-affected regions is nothing short of a major diplomatic success. If at all China deliberately hid facts or underreported the situation, as is alleged, it will be known to the world in due course when these international experts document their observations.

Why do we have to jump into conclusions without any evidence and tarnish the image of hardworking health workers who have been slogging day in out treating patients? Those leading the vitriol online attack against the WHO and its chief must answer if slander, malice and a hatred-filled anti-China campaign is how these tireless medicos deserve to be treated with for their services.

Priority right now should be to control the situation, not to embroil ourselves in mudslinging and waste our energy by pointing fingers in a show of one-upmanship. Investigations into who and what went wrong (if at all) can wait. Saving lives can't.

The other reason why the WHO and Dr Ghebreyesus are being attacked stems from the argument that Dr Ghebreyesus didn't declare coronavirus outbreak an international health emergency at an earlier date.

Those forwarding this argument must understand that decisions to declare an international emergency cannot be based on one person's whims and fancies. Far from being a one-person show, it involves rigorous assessments and deliberations between various stakeholders, all of which takes time. Even before declaring it an international health emergency, the WHO had been rigorously following up on research and treatment of coronavirus patients in China.

However, none of this means China, the WHO or Dr Ghebreyesus are above questioning. One must question them by all means, but personal attacks and a campaign aimed at tarnishing individuals and maligning an entire country is definitely not the way to do so.

AUTHORITIES SILENCE NEWS OF OUTBREAK

On January 3, Chinese authorities summoned Li and seven other doctors and accused them of spreading rumours. A stern message calling for an end to rumour-mongering was broadcast across China. "The police call on all netizens to not fabricate rumours, not spread rumours, not believe rumours," the message read.

Li was made to sign an affidavit acknowledging his crime and had to promise he will not engage in any such activities in the future. But Li's troubles did not end there. The ophthalmologist returned to work soon. While treating a patient affected with coronavirus, the infection was also transmitted to Li. Over the coming days, he showed the same symptoms — coughing, shortness of breath and fever.

By January 12, he was admitted to a hospital. His condition continued to deteriorate and he had to be shifted to the ICU. It was not till January 20 that China would take stock of the spread of coronavirus and declare a national emergency. On the same day, Chinese President Xi Jinping said, "People's lives and health should be given top priority and the spread of the outbreak should be resolutely curbed."

Li's diagnosis of coronavirus was only confirmed on February 1. He died five days later.

Too Much Censorship Led To Virus Outbreak

A too-harsh crackdown on online rumours during China's deadly viral epidemic had undermined public trust, China's top court said in a highly rare rebuke of the police force. Supreme Court Judge Tang Xinghua wrote Wednesday that officers should have been more lenient with those informing of the outbreak.

If the public had believed these rumours' at the time, and carried out measures like wearing masks, strictly disinfecting and avoiding wildlife markets it might have been a good thing, he said. Wuhan police responded in a post on the social media platform Weibo that they had only given education and criticism to the eight and had not meted out harsher punishment such as warnings, fines, or detention. But some users were unhappy with the reply, with one demanding the police apologize and asking: Is it so hard to acknowledge you have done wrong? Authorities in Wuhan have already been criticized online for withholding information about the infection until the end of last year, despite knowing about the new illness weeks earlier.

CHINA CORONAVIRUS: A VISUAL GUIDE

A new respiratory virus first detected in the Chinese city of Wuhan has infected hundreds of Chinese citizens and claimed a number of lives. The fast-spreading infection, which causes pneumonia-like symptoms, has prompted Chinese authorities to quarantine several major cities and cancel some Lunar New Year events. Here are six maps and graphics that will help you understand what is going on.

Cases have been mainly in China

Hundreds of patients have been infected with the virus across China, with central

Hubei province the worst-affected. The World Health Organisation (WHO) is warning the number of cases is likely to rise further, and Chinese authorities have introduced a number of measures to try to halt the virus's spread.

Travel restrictions have been imposed on a number of cities in Hubei province and people have been asked to wear face masks in public places. The Chinese government has also closed a number of temples, the Forbidden City and part of the Great Wall. The growing list of restrictions comes at the beginning of a week-long holiday celebrating Lunar New Year – one of the most important dates in the Chinese calendar – when millions of people travel home.

The WHO has not yet classed the virus as an "international emergency", partly because of the low number of overseas cases, but said it "may yet become one". "Make no mistake, this is, though, an emergency in China," said WHO director-general Dr. Tedros Adhanom Ghebreyesus.

Hubei province has been particularly badly affected

More than 500 cases have been recorded in Hubei province – the centre of the virus outbreak. Restrictions on travel are affecting at least 20 million people across 10 cities – including the capital Wuhan, where the virus emerged.

Its origins have been linked to the city's seafood market. Wuhan – which has a population of 11 million people – has gone into lockdown, with authorities suspending flights and train services in and out of the city.

"My university is checking every student's body temperature every day and are offering free masks. It also has its own hospital and ambulance," Chongthan Pepe Bifhowjit, an Indian student at the Wuhan University of Technology, told the BBC.

In a bid to tackle the increased demand for medical services, the authorities are building a new 1,000-bed hospital in the capital. State-owned news outlet Changjiang Daily said the hospital could be ready by 3 February. A total of 35 diggers and 10 bulldozers are currently working on the site.

There have been some cases elsewhere

Outside China, confirmed cases have been recorded in Thailand, Vietnam, Taiwan, South Korea, Singapore, Nepal, Japan, the US and France. Other nations are investigating suspected cases, including the UK and Canada.

Many authorities have announced screening measures for passengers from China, including the major airport hubs of Dubai and Abu Dhabi. Taiwan has banned people arriving from Wuhan, and the US state department warned its nationals to exercise increased caution in China.

The symptoms are respiratory

Coronaviruses are common, and typically cause mild respiratory symptoms, such as a cough or runny nose. But some are more serious – such as the deadly Sars (Severe Acute Respiratory Syndrome) and Middle East Respiratory Syndrome (Mers).

This outbreak – known as novel coronavirus (nCoV) – is a new strain that has not been previously identified in humans. It seems to start with a fever, followed by a dry cough and then, after a week, leads to shortness of breath. But in more severe cases, infection can cause pneumonia, severe acute respiratory syndrome, kidney failure and even death. Most victims have been elderly people, suffering from other chronic diseases including Parkinson's and diabetes.

Peter Piot, professor of global health and director of the London School of Hygiene & Tropical Medicine, said the "good news" was that data suggested the virus may have a lower mortality than Sars. There was also a diagnostic test and greater global sharing of information than previously, he said.

"And that is essential because you cannot deal with a potential pandemic in one country alone." There is not yet a specific anti-viral treatment for the infection, so people with the virus are currently being treated for their symptoms.

You can do things to reduce your chances of catching it

The WHO is advising people in affected areas to follow standard procedures to reduce the chance of catching the virus. They include hand and respiratory hygiene as well as safe food practices.

People are advised to avoid close contact with people suffering from acute respiratory infections; wash hands regularly, especially after direct contact with ill people or their environment; and avoid unprotected contact with farm or wild animals.

Avoiding eating raw or undercooked animal products is also advised. Those with symptoms of coronavirus should practise "cough etiquette", including maintaining distance, covering coughs and sneezes with disposable tissues or the inside of an elbow, and washing hands. The WHO has said that while there is evidence of transmission between people in close contact, such as families or those in healthcare settings, there is not yet evidence of onward transmission.

If a case is suspected, there are processes to follow

The Chinese government has classified the outbreak in the same category as the Sars epidemic. This means people diagnosed with the virus in the country must be isolated and can be placed in quarantine.

Within healthcare facilities, the WHO advises staff to implement enhanced standard infection prevention and control practices in hospitals, especially in emergency departments. The WHO advises that patients should be assessed quickly and treated for the level of severity of the disease they have – mild, moderate, or severe.

It also recommends immediately implementing infection prevention measures. These include staff wearing protective clothing and limiting patient movement around the hospital. In the UK, family doctors – GPs – are being advised to place patients suspected of having coronavirus in isolation and avoid physical examinations.

Official guidance from Public Health England (PHE) says patients should remain in a room away from other patients and staff and be prevented from using communal toilets. The UK government's emergency committee, Cobra, has held a meeting to discuss the outbreak.

THE SYMPTOMS ARE RESPIRATORY

Coronaviruses are common, and typically cause mild respiratory conditions, such as a cough or runny nose. But some are more serious - such as the deadly Sars and Mers - Middle East respiratory syndrome.

Covid-19 is a new strain not previously identified in humans. It seems to start with a fever, followed by a dry cough and leads to shortness of breath after a week.

Symptoms of China coronavirus

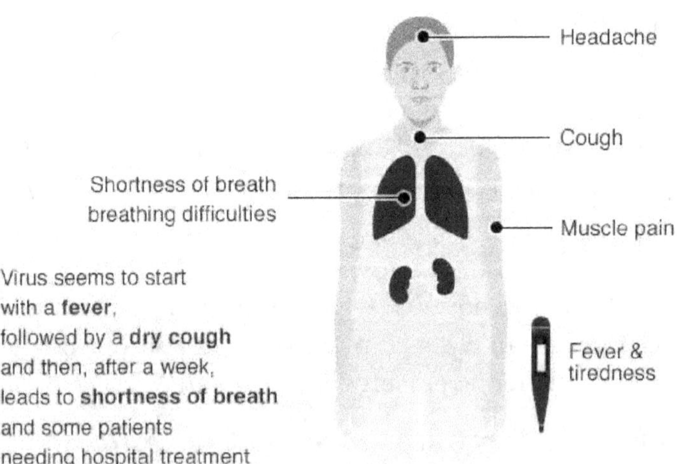

But in more severe cases, infection can cause pneumonia, severe acute respiratory syndrome, kidney failure and even death. A report on the early stages of the outbreak by the Lancet medical journal said most patients who died from the virus had had pre-existing conditions.

Medical researchers and scientists say it is too early to accurately predict how the virus will spread or calculate the death rate, partly due to mild cases remaining untested and unrecorded and a time lag of reporting infections.

There is not yet a specific anti-viral treatment for coronavirus, so people with the infection are currently being treated for their symptoms. The existence of coronavirus was first flagged by a Chinese doctor in late December, but he was reprimanded by local police for "spreading rumours".

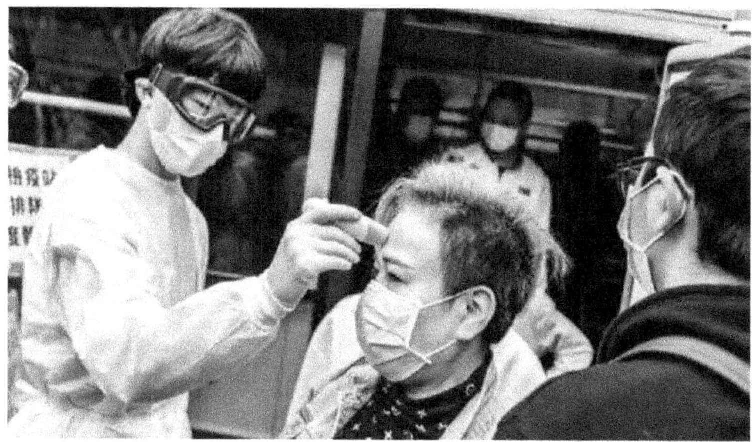

Dr Li Wenliang, a 34-year-old ophthalmologist, has since died from the illness. His death was met with an intense outpouring of grief on Chinese social media as well as anger towards Chinese authorities.

WHAT IS CORONAVIRUS AND WHAT ARE THE SYMPTOMS?

A virus causing severe lung disease that started in China has spread to 27 other countries, including the UK.

The coronavirus had infected 75,543 people in China as of 21 February, with 2,238 of them dying. What are the symptoms? It seems to start with a fever, followed by a dry cough.

After a week, it leads to shortness of breath and some patients require hospital treatment. Notably, the infection rarely seems to cause a runny nose or sneezing. The incubation period - between infection and showing any symptoms - lasts up to 14 days, according to the World Health Organization (WHO).

But some researchers say it may be as long as 24 days. And Chinese scientists say some people may be infectious even before their symptoms appear.

How deadly is the coronavirus? Based on data from 44,000 patients with this coronavirus, the WHO says:

- 81% develop mild symptoms
- 14% develop severe symptoms
- 5% become critically ill

The proportion dying from the disease, which has been named Covid-19, appears low (between 1% and 2%) - but the figures are unreliable. Thousands are still being treated but may go on to die - so the death rate could be higher.

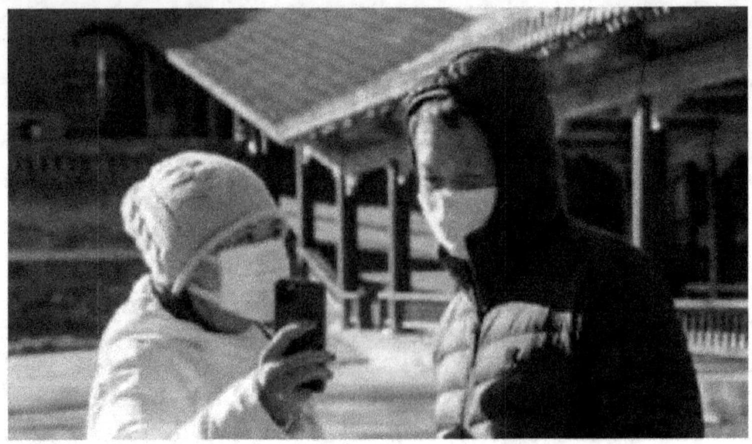

But it is also unclear how many mild cases remain unreported - so the death rate could also be lower. To put this it into context, about one billion people catch influenza every year, with between 290,000 and 650,000 deaths. The severity of flu changes every year.

Can coronavirus be treated or cured? Right now, treatment relies on the basics - keeping the patient's body going, including breathing support, until their immune system can fight off the virus.

However, the work to develop a vaccine is under way and it is hoped there will be human trials before the end of the year. Hospitals are also testing anti-viral drugs to see if they have an impact. How can I protect myself? The WHO says:

- Wash your hands - soap or hand gel can kill the virus
- Cover your mouth and nose when coughing or sneezing - ideally with a tissue - and wash your hands afterwards, to prevent the virus spreading
- Avoid touching your eyes, nose and mouth - if your hands touch a surface contaminated by the virus, this could transfer it into your body
- Don't get too close to people coughing, sneezing or with a fever - they can propel small droplets containing the virus into the air - ideally, keep 1m (3ft) away

How fast is it spreading ? Thousands of new cases are being reported each day. However, analysts believe the true scale could be 10 times larger than official figures.

China, where the outbreak began, has seen a sharp drop in the number of new infections. There were 394 new confirmed cases and 114 deaths reported on Wednesday, down from 1,749 new cases on Tuesday, the National Health Commission said.

The WHO says the outbreak, which it has declared a global emergency, can be contained. But some experts, including a former head of the US Centers for Disease Control, say it could become a pandemic - a global epidemic.

It's highly likely that #2019nCov will be a #pandemic, spreading beyond #China. We don't know yet whether the pandemic will be mild, moderate or severe. Key is to find and implement the best ways to protect people. With colds and flu tending to spread fastest in the winter, there is hope the turning of the seasons may help stem the outbreak.

School holidays may also help to slow its spread. However, a different strain of coronavirus - Middle East respiratory syndrome - emerged in the summer, in Saudi Arabia, so there's no guarantee warmer weather will halt the outbreak.

How did it start? This virus is not really "new" - it is just new to humans, having jumped from one species to another. Many of the early cases were linked to the South China Seafood Wholesale Market, in Wuhan. In China, a lot of people come into close contact with animals harbouring viruses - and the country's dense urban population means the disease can be easily spread.

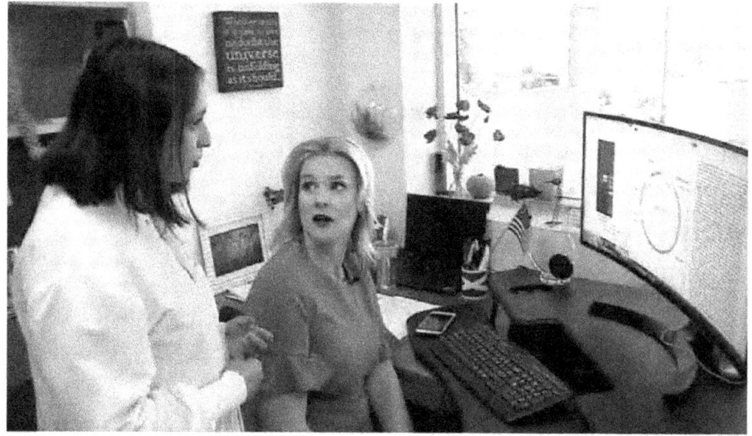

Media captionInside the US laboratory developing a coronavirus vaccine

Severe acute respiratory syndrome (Sars), which is also caused by a coronavirus, started off in bats and then infected the civet cat, which in turn passed it on to humans. The Sars outbreak, which started in China in 2002, killed 774 of the 8,098 people infected. The current virus - one of seven types of coronavirus - does not seem to be mutating so far. But while it appears stable, this is something scientists will be watching closely.

CORONAVIRUS: ALL YOU NEED TO KNOW ABOUT SYMPTOMS AND RISKS

According to the WHO, coronaviruses are a family of viruses that cause illnesses ranging from the common cold to more severe diseases such as severe acute respiratory syndrome (SARS) and the Middle East respiratory syndrome (MERS). These viruses were originally transmitted between animals and people. SARS, for instance, was transmitted from civet cats to humans while MERS moved to humans from a type of camel. Several known coronaviruses are circulating in animals that have not yet infected humans.

The name coronavirus comes from the Latin word corona, meaning crown or halo. Under an electron microscope, the image of the virus looks like a solar corona. The novel coronavirus, identified by Chinese authorities on January 7 and since named COVID-19, is a new strain that had not been previously identified in humans. Little is known about it, although human-to-human transmission has been confirmed.

What are the symptoms ?

According to the WHO, signs of infection include fever, cough, shortness of breath and breathing difficulties. In more severe cases, it can lead to pneumonia, multiple organ failure and even death.

Current estimates of the incubation period - the amount of time between infection and the onset of symptoms - range from one to 14 days. Most infected people show symptoms within five to six days.

However, infected patients can also be asymptomatic, meaning they do not display any symptoms despite having the virus in their systems.

How deadly is it? With more than 2,442 recorded deaths, the number of fatalities from this new coronavirus has surpassed the toll of the 2002-2003 SARS outbreak, which also originated in China.

SARS killed about 9 percent of those it infected - nearly 800 people worldwide and more than 300 in China alone. MERS, which did not spread as widely, was more deadly, killing one-third of those it infected. While the new coronavirus is more widespread in China than SARS in terms of case numbers, the mortality rate remains considerably lower at approximately 2 percent, according to the WHO.

Where have cases been reported? Most cases and deaths have been reported in China - the vast majority in Hubei province.

Deaths have also been confirmed in Hong Kong, the Philippines, Japan, France, Taiwan, South Korea, Italy and Iran. The virus has spread to many countries in the Asia-Pacific region as well as in Europe, North America, the Middle East and Africa. The majority of cases outside China are among people who recently travelled to the country, however instances of human-to-human transmission have been recorded in several countries and questions have been raised about cases with no apparent link to China.

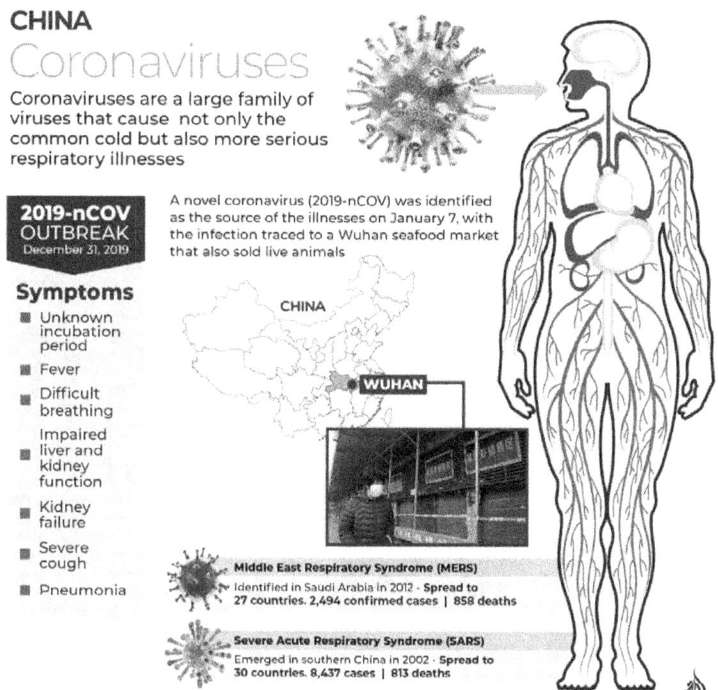

What is being done to stop it from spreading? Scientists around the globe are racing to develop a vaccine but have warned that one is unlikely to be available for mass distribution before 2021. Meanwhile, Chinese authorities have effectively sealed off Wuhan and placed restrictions on travel to and from several other cities, affecting some 60 million people.

Many international airlines have cancelled flights to China. Some countries have banned Chinese nationals from entering their territories and several more have evacuated their citizens from Wuhan. Where did the virus originate? Chinese health authorities are still trying to determine the origin of the virus, which they say likely came from a seafood market in Wuhan where wildlife was also traded illegally.

On February 7, Chinese researchers said the virus could have spread from an infected animal species to humans through illegally-trafficked pangolins, which are prized in Asia for food and medicine. Scientists have pointed to either bats or snakes as the source of the virus.

The decision to sound the top-level alarm was made after the first cases of human-to-human transmission outside China were confirmed. The international health alert is a call to countries around the world to coordinate their response under the guidance of the United Nations health agency.

There have been five global health emergencies since 2005 when the declaration was formalised: swine flu in 2009, polio in 2014, Ebola in 2014, Zika in 2016 and Ebola again in 2019.

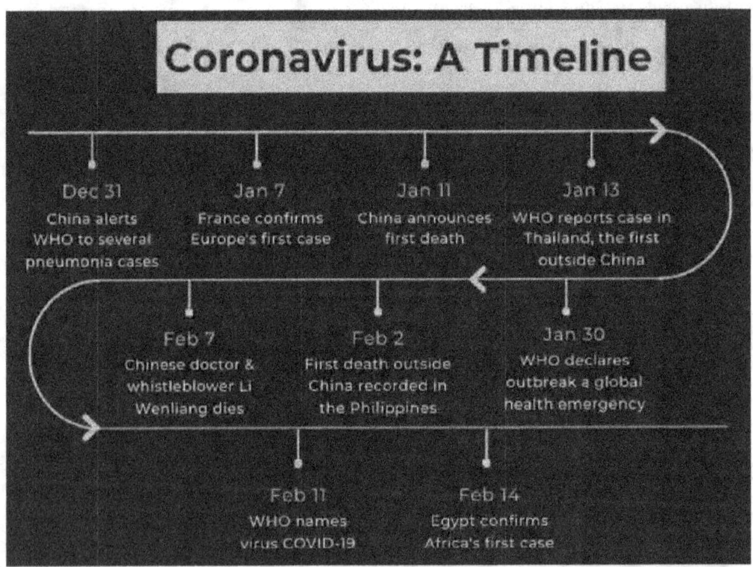

Is this a global emergency? The outbreak now constitutes a global health emergency, the WHO said on January 30.

CORONAVIRUS EXPLAINED: WHAT YOU NEED TO KNOW

A new Chinese coronavirus, a cousin of the SARS virus, has infected hundreds since the outbreak began in Wuhan, China, in December. Scientist Leo Poon, who first decoded the virus, thinks it likely started in an animal and spread to humans. "What we know is it causes pneumonia and then doesn't respond to antibiotic treatment, which is not surprising, but then in terms of mortality, SARS kills 10% of the individuals," Poon, a virologist at the School of Public Health at The University of Hong Kong, said. It's not clear how deadly the Wuhan coronavirus will be, but fatality rates are currently lower than both MERS and SARS. Experts stress that it will change as the outbreak develops.

China confirms new coronavirus can spread between humans

The World Health Organization offered guidance to countries on how they can prepare for it, including how to monitor for the sick and how to treat patients. Here's what you should know about coronaviruses. What is a coronavirus? Coronaviruses are a large group of viruses that are common among animals. In rare cases, they are what scientists call zoonotic, meaning they can be transmitted from animals to humans, according to the US Centers for Disease Control and Prevention.

Coronavirus symptoms

The viruses can make people sick, usually with a mild to moderate upper respiratory tract illness, similar to a common cold. Coronavirus symptoms include a runny nose, cough, sore throat, possibly a headache and maybe a fever, which can last for a couple of days.

For those with a weakened immune system, the elderly and the very young, there's a chance the virus could cause a lower, and much more serious, respiratory tract illness like a pneumonia or bronchitis.

There are a handful of human coronaviruses that are known to be deadly. Middle East respiratory syndrome, also known as the MERS virus, was first reported in the Middle East in 2012 and also causes respiratory problems, but those symptoms are much more severe. Three to four out of every 10 patients infected with MERS died, according to the CDC.

Severe acute respiratory syndrome, also known as SARS, is the other coronavirus that can cause more severe symptoms. First identified in the Guangdong province in southern China, according to the WHO, it causes respiratory problems but can also cause diarrhea, fatigue, shortness of breath, respiratory distress and kidney failure.

Depending on the patient's age, the death rate with SARS ranged from 0-50% of the cases, with older people being the most vulnerable.

The Wuhan coronavirus is currently thought to be more mild than SARS and MERS and takes longer to develop symptoms. Patients to date have typically experienced a mild cough for a week followed by shortness of breath, causing them to visit the hospital, explains Peter Horby, professor of emerging infectious diseases and global health at the University of Oxford. So far, around 15% to 20% of cases have become severe, requiring, for example, ventilation in the hospital.

How it spreads

Viruses can spread from human contact with animals. Scientists think MERS started in camels, according to the WHO. With SARS, scientists suspected civet cats were to blame. Officials do not yet know what animal may have caused the current outbreak in Wuhan.

When it comes to human-to-human transmission of the viruses, often it happens when someone comes into contact with an infected person's secretions, such as droplets in a cough.

Depending on how virulent the virus is, a cough, sneeze or handshake could cause exposure. The virus can also be transmitted by touching something an infected person has touched and then touching your mouth, nose or eyes. Caregivers can sometimes be exposed by handling a patient's waste, according to the CDC.

Human-to-human transmission has been confirmed for the Wuhan coronavirus, but experts are now trying to understand who is transmitting it most, who is at most risk and whether transmission is occurring mostly in hospitals or in the community. SARS and MERS were largely transmitted inside hospitals, Horby said. Some people are also considered to be "superspreaders."

Who is affected? MERS, SARS and the Wuhan coronavirus appear to cause more severe disease in older people, though uncertainty remains around the latest outbreak. Of the cases of Wuhan coronavirus reported so far, none are yet confirmed to be among children, Horby said. The average age is people 40 or over, he said.

Coronavirus treatment

There is no specific treatment, but research is underway. Most of the time, symptoms will go away on their own and experts advise seeking care early. If symptoms feel worse than a standard cold, see your doctor. Doctors can relieve symptoms by prescribing a pain or fever medication. The CDC says a room humidifier or a hot shower can help with a sore throat or cough.

Drink plenty of fluids, get rest and sleep as much as possible. Should you worry about the Wuhan coronavirus? The Wuhan coronavirus fatality rate is lower than for SARS and MERS, but still comparable to the 1918 Spanish flu pandemic, explains Neil Ferguson, professor of mathematical biology at Imperial College London.

"It is a significant concern, globally," Ferguson says, noting that we don't fully understand the severity. Ferguson believes the fatality rate is likely to be lower due to an "iceberg" of milder cases we are yet to find, but he highlights that novel viruses spread much faster through a population.

How can you can prevent it? There is no vaccine to protect against this family of viruses, at least not yet. Trials for a MERS vaccine are underway. The US National Institutes of Health is working on a vaccine against the new virus, but it will be months until clinical trials get underway and more than a year until it might become available.

You may be able to reduce your risk of infection by avoiding people who are sick. Try to avoid touching your eyes, nose and mouth.

Wash your hands often with soap and water and for at least 20 seconds. Awareness is key. If you are sick and have reason to believe it may be the Wuhan coronavirus due to travel to the region or coming into contact with someone who has been there, you should let a health care provider know and seek treatment early.

Cover your mouth and nose when you cough or sneeze, and disinfect the objects and surfaces you touch. If traveling to China, be aware of symptoms and avoid live animal markets, which is where the latest outbreak began in Wuhan.

Coronavirus and pregnancy

In pregnant women, the more severe versions of MERS and SARS coronaviruses can be serious. There are cases in which a woman infected with MERS had a stillbirth, a 2014 study showed. SARS-associated illnesses were linked to cases of spontaneous abortion, maternal death and critical maternal illness, a 2004 study found.

Coronavirus and cats, dogs and other animals

Pets can catch coronaviruses and the infections can become severe. Sometimes the viruses can lead to deadly diseases. One can cause feline infectious peritonitis in cats and something called a pantropic canine coronavirus can infect cats and dogs, according to a 2011 study.

Cats can catch SARS, but none of the infected cats developed symptoms, according to the study. The feline coronavirus typically is asymptomatic, but can cause mild diarrhea. Feline infectious peritonitis, or FIP, can cause flu-like symptoms for a cat, but can also be more serious for cats and can cause organ failure, but it is not contagious and will not spread from animal to animal or person to person.

RESEARCH FINDS NEW WAYS COVID-19 CAN BE SPREAD

The COVID-19 outbreak continues to spread in China and worldwide, with more than 76,000 total confirmed cases and deaths topping 2,200. Researchers are studying how those infected shed the virus and what impact it's having on affected populations.

One new study has found answers that many won't find comforting. Testing and confirmation of novel coronavirus infection is currently carried out by oral swabs. But research published Feb. 17 in Emerging Microbes & Infections finds evidence that there's an oral-fecal transmission route.

The scientists reported that COVID-19 genetic material was detected in both anal swabs and blood samples. "We detected the virus in oral swabs, anal swabs, and blood, thus infected patients can potentially shed this pathogen through respiratory, fecal-oral, or body fluid routes," the study authors wrote.

Chinese researchers conducted the study in a Wuhan, China hospital, and analyzed samples collected from about 180 patients. Crucially, evidence of COVID-19 was found in anal swabs and blood — even when it wasn't detected using oral swabs. According to the study, this was particularly true for those patients receiving supportive care for several days.

Findings also suggest that timing is an important factor. On day one of the illness, 80 percent of oral swabs were COVID-19 positive, but by day five, 75 percent of anal swabs were positive, while only half of the oral swabs showed infection, according to the study.

"These results confirm that COVID-19 patients have live virus in stool specimens, which is a new finding in the transmission routes of 2019-nCoV," wrote authors of a study, published by the Chinese Centers for Disease Control (CCDC) publication, CCDC Weekly. This means that sneezing isn't the only way to spread this infection; blood and fecal matter can carry the virus, even when conventional testing comes back negative.

"The virus can also be transmitted through the potential fecal-oral route. This means that stool samples may contaminate hands, food, water, etc., and may cause infection by invading the oral cavity, respiratory mucosa, conjunctiva, etc," study authors concluded.

Coronavirus study finds who's most at risk

Although medical staff, people with illnesses, and older adults are most at risk, more than 80 percent of COVID-19 cases have been mild, according to a new report from the Chinese Center for Disease Control and Prevention (China CDC).

The Hubei province in China, where the infection is believed to have originated, is the hardest hit, according to the report. The province's death rate is almost 3 percent, compared with just under a half percent in the rest of the country. In the United States, 13 Americans who were evacuated from the Diamond Princess cruise ship on U.S. charter flights are being tested and treated for COVID-19, according to the University of Nebraska Medical Center.

They'll be held in the new National Quarantine Unit, which was designed to safely monitor Americans after exposure to an infectious disease. The unit is nearby the Nebraska Biocontainment Unit Team, which cared for three people who contracted Ebola in 2014.

"We were there for Ebola, we were there for the rescued Americans now being monitored at Camp Ashland, and we're going to be there for these American citizens as well," said Dr. Jeffrey P. Gold, chancellor of the University of Nebraska Medical Center and University of Nebraska at Omaha, in a statement. These 13 evacuees join the 15 other Americans who have received a diagnosis of COVID-19.

On Tuesday, 346 Americans who were evacuated from Wuhan, China amid the coronavirus outbreak have left quarantine at two California military bases, according to NPR.

CDC director warns COVID-19 may spread throughout U.S.

COVID-19, the extremely infectious coronavirus sweeping through China's Hubei province, will become a 'community virus' in the United States, if not this year, then the next, CDC director Dr. Robert Redfield told CNN Feb. 13. "This virus is probably with us beyond this season, beyond this year, and I think eventually the virus will find a foothold and we will get community-based transmission," said Dr. Redfield. "Right now we're in an aggressive containment mode."

Dr. Redfield emphasized that the CDC doesn't have any evidence that coronavirus is "really embedded in the community at this time, but with that said, we want to intensify our surveillance so that we're basing those conclusions based on data." Alarmingly, one of the more concerning aspects of the COVID-19 coronavirus is that someone infected can transmit it when they have no obvious symptoms of infection.

"There's been good communication with our colleagues to confirm asymptomatic infection, to confirm asymptomatic transmission, to be able to get a better handle on the clinical spectrum of illness in China. What we don't know though is how much of the asymptomatic cases are driving transmission," Dr. Redfield confirmed.

On the Chinese mainland, over 1,700 medical workers have confirmed COVID-19 infections. World Health Organization (WHO) officials are working with Chinese authorities to find out when the health workers were infected with the coronavirus, and to determine if they were exposed to the virus unknowingly within a clinical environment and if they were wearing protective equipment at that time.

U.S. military prepares for pandemic, CDC warns further spread likely

U.S. military forces have been told to prepare for a possible pandemic situation due to the coronavirus virus, COVID-19, according to recently issued Navy and Marine Corps service-wide messages. The bulletin emphasized, "An outbreak of new (novel) coronavirus is rapidly evolving [but] currently poses a low risk to personnel located in CONUS [contiguous United States]."

Meanwhile, the WHO is rallying the international community to act rapidly. "The first vaccine could be ready in 18 months, so we have to do everything today using the available weapons to fight this virus, while preparing for the long-term," said WHO director-general, Tedros Ghebreyesus in a statement. "You strike hard when the window of opportunity is there. That's what we're saying to the rest of the world."

Last week there was a huge jump in new cases, almost 15,000 in the Hubei province (the epicenter of the outbreak). But the increase is due to a change in the criteria for counting diagnoses of the virus.

Hubei had previously only used RNA tests to confirm infection, which can take days to process, delaying treatment. Now, CT scans are being used to reveal lung infection, which can speed up treatment to improve the chances of recovery, according to a New York Times report.

Domestically, another case of COVID-19 was confirmed in Texas, according to the CDC. "The patient is among a group of people under a federal quarantine order at JBSA-Lackland in Texas because of their recent return to the U.S. on a State Department-chartered flight that arrived on February 7, 2020," the CDC announced in a statement.

Issues found in coronavirus tests fast-tracked by FDA

Officials from the CDC reported issues with tests designed to detect if someone is infected with the new coronavirus. Dr. Nancy Messonnier, director of the National Center for Immunization and Respiratory Diseases, said in a press conference Feb. 12Trusted Source that the tests were sent out to different states and at least 30 countries. As part of routine testing, issues were discovered with the tests called a 2019-nCoV Real-Time RT-PCR Diagnostic Panel. "The states identified some inconclusive laboratory results," she explained. "We are working closely with them to correct the issues."

Messonnier said that replacement materials would be sent out for states that reported issues. "Speed is important, but equally or more important in this situation is making sure the laboratory results are correct," she said.

The Food and Drug Administration (FDA) issued an emergency authorization on Feb. 4 allowing public health labs to use the test that can detect whether someone is infected with the new coronavirus. This authorization was especially significant for the United States because hospitals and public health departments were in theory able to conduct testing on-site rather than shipping virus samples directly to the CDC. Until these issues are fixed, local medical officials will still have to send samples to the CDC.

The deadly virus gets a new name

The WHO announced on Feb. 11 that the new coronavirus originating in China would now be called COVID-19. Previously, it had been called 2019nCoV, although many media outlets referred to the virus simply as coronavirus, even though that refers to a larger family of viruses.

WHO chief says spreading outside of China may be 'tip of the iceberg'

The director-general of the WHO warned that the international community should prepare for the spread of the novel coronavirus to accelerate. "There've been some concerning instances of onward 2019nCoV spread from people with no travel history to [China]. The detection of a small number of cases may indicate more widespread transmission in other countries; in short, we may only be seeing the tip of the iceberg," tweeted Tedros Ghebreyesus, director-general of WHO on Feb. 9.

A cruise ship in Japan has been quarantined as hundreds of the 3,700 passengers were found to be infected with the virus. "Our guests and crew onboard Diamond Princess are the focus of our entire global organization right now and all of our hearts are with each of them," said Jan Swartz, Princess Cruises president in a statement.

Ghebreyesus emphasized that, "In an evolving public health emergency, all countries must step up efforts to prepare for 2019nCoV's possible arrival and do their utmost to contain it should it arrive. This means lab capacity for rapid diagnosis, contact tracing and other tools in the public health arsenal."

However, "dramatic reductions" in the pace of the disease's spread should begin this month if containment works, said Dr. Ian Lipkin, director of Columbia University's Center for Infection and Immunity on Feb. 9, according to AP News.

NIAID director discusses latest developments

The virus is likely to continue spreading in the United States, the CDC said.

The National Institute of Allergies and Infectious Diseases (NIAID) director, Dr. Anthony Fauci, discussed the ongoing novel coronavirus epidemic in a livestream video Feb. 6 with Journal of the American Medical Association (JAMA) editor in chief, Dr. Howard Bauchner.

"One thing is starting to be noticed. It appears that the travel-related cases that are outside of China, that then transmit to other people, it appears that somehow or other not a lot of them are catastrophic infection," observed Fauci.

Fauci also doesn't believe that current restrictions on travel will be effective to contain the outbreak, because they "don't do much to stop the entry of infection when there is a broad, global pandemic, because you can't restrict travel for the whole world."

Fauci also told JAMA that the novel coronavirus, unlike other infections, can take a long time after infection to cause severe illness. "This virus is really acting different. This virus, when it gets in you, it adapts itself so that you can wind up days later getting really serious disease," emphasized Fauci.

WHO declares emergency

The WHO announced that it's declaring a public health emergency of international concern based on the outbreak of the new coronavirus. Dr. Tedros Adhanom Ghebreyesus, WHO director-general, said at a press conference that they were concerned about the virus' ability to spread outside of China.

"The main resound or the declaration is not because of what is happening but because of what is happening in other continues. The greatest concern is the potential for the virus to spread to countries with weaker systems... that are ill-prepared to deal with it," Ghebreyesus said. Person-to-person transmission has been seen among people in contact with those who have the virus.

The full picture of how easily and sustainably this coronavirus spreads is still unclear. Person-to-person transmission can happen on a continuum, with some viruses being highly contagious (like measles) and others being less so. "This is a very serious public health situation," said Dr. Nancy Messonnier, director of the National Center for Immunization and Respiratory Diseases, in an earlier statement. "Moving forward, we can expect to see more cases, and more cases means more potential for person-to-person spread," she said.

FDA announces new countermeasures against Wuhan virus

The FDA will take critical actions to advance countermeasures against the new coronavirus, the administration announced on Jan. 27.

"We have a vital mission to protect and promote public health and the FDA is closely collaborating with our domestic and international public health partners to mitigate the impact of the novel coronavirus that emerged in Wuhan, China," said FDA Commissioner Stephen M. Hahn, MD, in a statementTrusted Source.

The news comes amid a significant increase in reported infections. Hahn emphasized the FDA will begin employing the full range of the administration's public health employees to "facilitate the development and availability of investigational medical products to help address this urgent public health situation."

The FDA has also launched a landing pageTrusted Source that provides "key information for the public, including product developers, on the FDA's efforts in response to this outbreak."

This outbreak is affecting healthy and relatively young people as well, according to a recent studyTrusted Source published in The Lancet. The researchers also found that most cases may be very mild, facilitating a more rapid transmission of the epidemic.

Crucially, only two-thirds of the 41 patients studied had visited the Wuhan seafood market. The most common symptoms at onset of illness were fever, cough, and muscle pain or fatigue, according to study authors.

"It is expected that further international exportation of cases may appear in any country. Thus, all countries should be prepared for containment, including active surveillance, early detection, isolation and case management, contact tracing, and prevention of onward spread of 2019-nCoV infection, and to share full data with WHO," the World Health Organization said in a statementTrusted Source.

Level 3 health warning issued for Wuhan by CDC

On Jan. 23, the CDC escalated its health warning regarding travel to Wuhan, China, to a level 3. This means the CDC advises travelers to avoid nonessential travel to Wuhan, China — previously identified as the epicenter of the recent outbreak.

According to the CDC:

- Chinese officials have closed transport in and out of Wuhan, including buses, subways, trains, and the international airport.

- Preliminary information suggests older adults and people with underlying health conditions may be at increased risk for severe disease from this virus.
- Person-to-person transmission has been confirmed.

Officials admitted they don't know the source of this virus, and "we don't understand how easily it spreads and we don't fully understand its clinical features or severity."

According to a report in China state media, tighter regulations will be imposed on vehicles leaving the city.

Additionally, vehicles are banned from taking passengers out of Wuhan, and measures including body temperature monitoring of drivers and vehicle disinfection will be implemented.

Another MERS and SARS?

According to the WHOTrusted Source, initial information about the pneumonia cases in Wuhan, provided by Chinese authorities, pointed to the coronavirus as the pathogen causing this cluster.

Chinese authorities reported that laboratory tests ruled out SARS-CoV, MERS-CoV, influenza, avian influenza, adenovirus, and other common infectious agents.

More than 8,000 people contracted the SARS virus, and almost 800 died in the 2002 pandemic.

The SARS virus spread to nearly 40 countriesTrusted Source in 2002 and 2003. The same type of virus was associated with a similar outbreak of MERS, which was first identified in 2013 Trusted Source in Saudi Arabia. According to the WHOTrusted Source, MERS has been responsible for about 850 deaths worldwide.

Coronaviruses are a large family of viruses, with some causing less severe disease, like the common cold. Although some easily transmit from person to person, others don't.

Infection linked to local food market

China state media reported that some of the people who fell ill between Dec. 12 and 29 are sellers from a local wholesale seafood market.

That market has since been shut down for cleaning and disinfection, according to the CDC.

"What's happening over there is in a particular area of China at a seafood market, and... it [first] appears that transmission is from animal to human," Nikhil Bhayani, an infectious disease physician with Texas Health Resources, told Healthline.

What is a coronavirus?

"Corona means 'crown,' so these viruses appear crown-shaped when looked at under an electron microscope," said Bhanu Sud, MD, an infectious disease specialist at St. Jude Medical Center in Placentia, California.

"Most coronaviruses are harmless," he said. "They'll usually cause mild to moderate upper respiratory tract illnesses, like the common cold. Most people will get infected with these viruses at some point in their lives."

Sud emphasizes that while the outlook is good for most people infected with this type of virus, the SARS and MERS strains are more serious.

The death rate is around 10 percent for people with SARS and 30 percent for those with the MERS variant.

"What is unknown right now is the virus being typed. They're doing testing to find out what type of virus this is and whether it's more similar to SARS or MERS," Bhayani said. "I have a strong feeling that this is going to be a new virus."

Chinese authorities turn to quarantines to stop the outbreak

China has started to shut down flights and trains from Wuhan, effectively quarantining a city of millions, according to reports.

According to an earlier translated report from the Wuhan Municipal Health Commission:

"Experts advise that the city is currently in the season of high incidence of infectious diseases in winter and spring. Citizens should pay attention to maintaining indoor air circulation, avoiding closed and airless public places and crowded places, and wear masks if necessary."

Sud said, "Any infection anywhere in the world is always a risk for every country because international travel has become so easy now."

He adds this is why early detection and quarantine are essential measures in halting the transmission of these infections.

No treatment available

According to Sud, human coronaviruses most commonly transmit from an infected person to others via:

- the air by coughing and sneezing
- close personal contact, such as touching or shaking hands
- touching an object or surface with the virus on it, then touching your mouth, nose, or eyes before washing your hands

"In the United States, people usually get infected with common human coronaviruses in the fall and winter. However, infection can occur at any time of the year," he said.

"Most people will get infected with one or more of the common human coronaviruses in their lifetime," he added.

Sud also points out both SARS and MERS outbreaks were from animal-to-human contact, with SARS most likely from contact with bats and MERS from contact with camels.

"Since the organism causing infection is a virus, to date, we don't have any specific antiviral medications," Sud said.

The bottom line

Chinese authorities have identified an outbreak of respiratory illness. The CDC has issued a level 3 warning due to the outbreak, notifying travelers they should avoid nonessential travel to the area.

So far, 15 people in the United States have been confirmed to have contracted the new coronavirus.

Experts emphasize that since a virus causes the illness, there aren't any treatments available. The infection can only be allowed to run its course.

WE KNOW ABOUT THE CORONAVIRUS, FROM SYMPTOMS TO WHO IS AT RISK

Concern is high about a dangerous new coronavirus behind an epidemic in China and illnesses in 26 other countries. The number of people sick with or dying of a viral pneumonia caused by the virus is still rising in the epicenter of Hubei Province, China, despite a quarantine of some 60 million people and other measures to stop it. International health officials are also worried about growing clusters of illness elsewhere, including among people who have neither been to China nor in contact with anyone who has. Most cases outside China were part of an outbreak on the Diamond Princess cruise ship in Japan. The epidemic has interrupted travel and business and disrupted supplies of some goods—including those needed to fight the epidemic.

Scientists and public-health officials are learning more all the time about the virus, called Severe Acute Respiratory Syndrome Coronavirus 2, or SARS-CoV-2. The disease it causes is called Covid-19.

Among key questions they are seeking answers to are how the virus is transmitted, how easily it spreads and how many people are infected but don't develop symptoms.

This new virus belongs to a family of viruses known as coronaviruses. Named for the crown-like spikes on their surfaces, they infect mostly bats, pigs and small mammals. But they mutate easily and can jump from animals to humans, and from one human to another. In recent years, they have become a growing player in infectious-disease outbreaks world-wide.

Seven strains are known to infect humans, including this new virus, causing illnesses in the respiratory tract. Four of those strains cause common colds. Two others, by contrast, rank among the deadliest of human infections: severe acute respiratory syndrome, or SARS, and Middle East respiratory syndrome, or MERS.

What are the symptoms of the illness and how do you know if you have it? The virus infects the lower respiratory tract. Patients initially develop a fever, cough and aches, and can progress to shortness of breath and complications from pneumonia, according to case reports. They might develop nausea, with vomiting and diarrhea. Some become only mildly ill, or are infected but don't get sick. Others are mildly ill for a few days, then rapidly develop more severe symptoms of pneumonia.

Some patients haven't had a fever initially or might develop a "walking pneumonia," meaning they might spread their infection to others because they aren't sick enough to be in a hospital.

Who is most at risk? Adults of all ages have been infected, but the risk is highest for older people and those with other health conditions such as diabetes. Most of the 1,023 people whose deaths were included in a study by the Chinese Center for Disease Control and Prevention were age 60 or older, and/or had other illnesses. Many patients who have died were admitted to hospitals when their illness was advanced. Few children have been reported with the infection, but that could change.

How at risk is someone in the U.S.? The risk to the U.S. public is low, says the U.S. Centers for Disease Control and Prevention. There are very few cases in the U.S., and the virus isn't spreading widely. The majority of confirmed infections are in people who were infected while abroad and were quarantined upon their return to the U.S. The CDC is monitoring for more cases through reports from health-care providers and local public health departments, surveillance systems and testing.

How is the virus spread among humans? It is likely spread through a cough, sneeze or other contact with saliva, Chinese officials say. There is no evidence of transmission by aerosol, or through the air. MERS and SARS spread mainly through "respiratory droplets" produced when someone coughs or sneezes. Those two viruses spread mostly through close contact.

Scientists are also investigating whether the new coronavirus may spread in feces, as tests have found it in the digestive tract of some patients.

What is the incubation period? People become ill between two and 14 days after infection, according to the U.S. CDC. Chinese researchers recently cited an average incubation period of 5.2 days.

Is there a test? Public-health officials have developed and are distributing diagnostic tests, which are being used to confirm whether a patient has the new coronavirus or another infection. In Hubei Province, cases are also being diagnosed based on chest X-rays and symptoms. Scientists are working on a blood test to detect antibodies to the virus, to determine how many people in the population have been infected. Some may not have gotten sick.

Can face masks protect you? Health experts and mask makers say only a properly used reusable N95 respirator mask certified by an independent agency can guard against the virus. Paper or polyurethane foam masks don't filter out smaller particles responsible for transmitting infectious agents. They may help prevent sick people from transmitting to others.

Touch

A coronavirus can also be transmitted by touching an object where airborne droplets have settled.

The viruses can survive briefly on surfaces depending on conditions of humidity and temperature.

Wearing a mask prevents direct contact with nose and mouth, and could protect a user who may have touched a contaminated area.

Masks

Frequently changing disposable masks, and washing your hands after, are important steps to avoid contamination from pathogens that cling to the outer surface.

N95 masks offer more protection. But they only work if they fit properly, and aren't suitable for children or people with facial hair. Surgical masks don't offer full protection against airborne viruses. They don't fully seal off the nose and mouth.

How easily does the new virus spread? Disease-modeling experts have estimated that on average, each infected person has transmitted the virus to about 2.6 others, though the range is between 1.5 and 3.5. Those rates are higher than for some influenza viruses, some are lower than SARS, and they are far lower than measles, in which one infected person can transmit the virus to 12 to 18 other people.

Public-health experts caution that these estimates are preliminary, change over time and can be lowered by measures to prevent the virus from spreading.

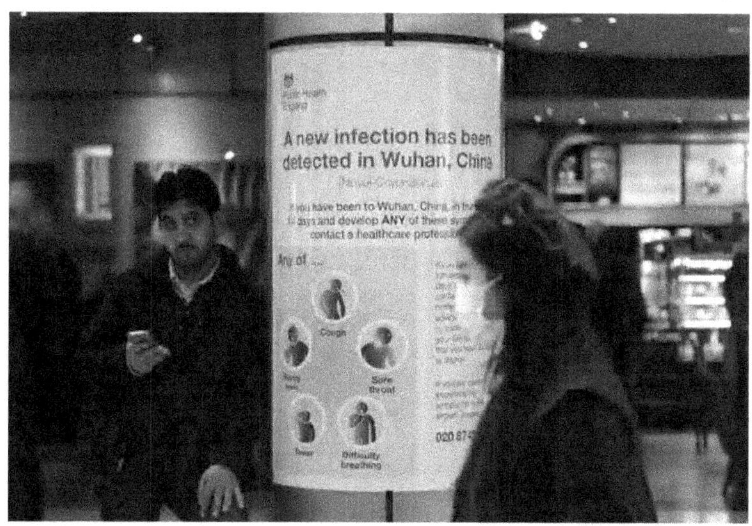

A Public Health England sign warns passengers at London's Heathrow Airport of the virus.

Can you catch the virus from someone even before they have symptoms? It is possible. But little is known so far. In Macau, a 15-year-old resident of Wuhan, the epicenter of the outbreak, tested positive for the coronavirus despite having no fever or cough, according to that special administrative region of China. Scientists reported in the Lancet medical journal that they identified the coronavirus in a 10-year-old boy who developed no symptoms, even though others in the child's family fell ill. Chinese news outlets have reported a handful of other potential asymptomatic cases.

Where did the new coronavirus come from? The new virus likely came originally from bats, scientists say. It isn't known exactly where or how it jumped to humans, though. Viruses from bats often infect another mammal first and then mutate to become more transmissible to humans. One hypothesis is that the intermediary animal for this new virus may be a pangolin, a small mammal sold in wildlife markets, prized for its meat and scales covering its body. Health officials believe the outbreak originated in a large animal and seafood market in Wuhan, China.

Of the first 41 cases, 27 had some exposure to that market, according to a report in the Lancet. But three of the first four people to become ill, on Dec. 1 and Dec. 10, said they had no contact with the market.

A study in the New England Journal of Medicine found that 55% of patients in Wuhan who became ill before Jan. 1 had a link to the market, compared with 8.6% of those who became ill after that point. Scientists say it will take some time to identify the exact source.

How dangerous is the new coronavirus: It appears to be less deadly than a related pathogen—SARS, which erupted in China in 2002 and spread globally in 2003. SARS killed about 10% of the people it infected, while about 2.9% of the people confirmed to be infected with this new coronavirus have died, according to World Health Organization data.

But the new virus spreads from one person to another more easily than SARS, some disease modeling and case studies suggest.

Is the virus mutating, particularly in a way that would make it more contagious? No. The virus has remained stable genetically thus far, according to the World Health Organization and the U.S. CDC.

Most people who are infected may become only mildly ill, data suggest. Of 44,672 cases in China, 81% had mild symptoms, 13.8% were severely ill, and 4.7% were critically ill, according to the Chinese CDC. All of those who died were in critical condition.

Public-health officials are trying to determine how many people have been infected, including those who didn't get sick at all. They are concerned and want to contain the virus because its effects aren't fully known. In addition, new viruses can mutate, possibly becoming more virulent as they work their way through a population.

Is it safe to travel to China? The U.S. State Department has warned Americans not to travel to China. Most commercial airlines have suspended or reduced flights to and from China. Americans who remain in China should stay home as much as possible, limit contact with others and follow guidelines from the U.S. Centers for Disease Control and Prevention to prevent infection, U.S. authorities say.

Is it safe to go on a cruise? The U.S. State Department has urged Americans to reconsider cruises to or within Asia, given the risk of infection and of being subjected to a lengthy quarantine.

Are there drugs to treat coronaviruses? There aren't any drugs or vaccines approved specifically for the new virus. But several are in development or being studied. Two clinical trials in China are evaluating remdesivir, an antiviral drug from Gilead Sciences Inc. that was also tested for Ebola. A hospital in Wuhan is conducting a clinical trial using a combination of two drugs for HIV that had been tested on MERS patients in Saudi Arabia. The therapy, sold under the brand name Kaletra in the U.S., is normally used to treat HIV patients and belongs to a class of drugs known as protease inhibitors, which block a key enzyme that helps viruses replicate. In addition, a few vaccine makers are developing products targeting the virus.

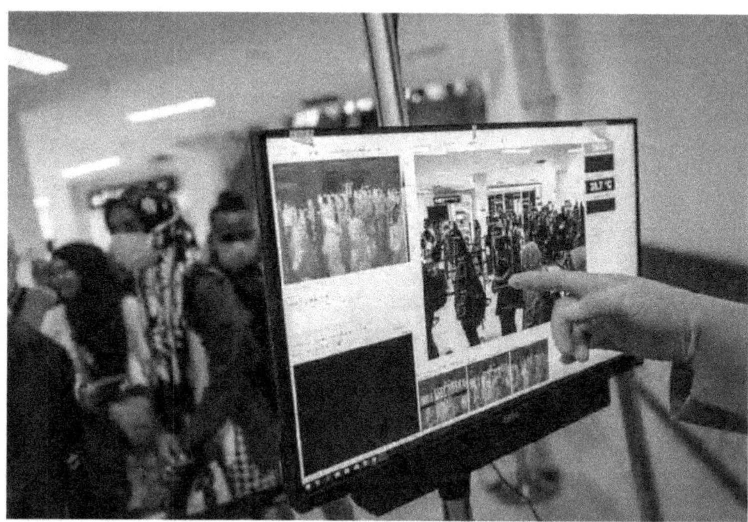

A health official watches travelers on a thermographic monitor at the Sultan Iskandar Muda International Airport in Indonesia.

What is being done to contain the spread of the virus? China imposed quarantines on Wuhan, the epicenter of the outbreak, and several other cities, affecting millions of citizens. Officials built a large field hospital in Wuhan to isolate and care for patients and are investigating chains of transmission. It isn't clear what effect the quarantine measures are having.

The U.S. imposed entry restrictions on foreign nationals who have visited China in the past 14 days. Most international airlines suspended flights from China. Americans who were evacuated from Hubei Province and a cruise ship where an outbreak occurred have undergone or are undergoing quarantines for 14 days.

There are few travelers from China currently. Those who do come to the U.S. are screened at the airport. Those who don't have symptoms of illness are asked to self-quarantine for 14 days.

Could goods imported from China carry the virus? That is unlikely, the CDC says. Coronaviruses generally don't survive long on inanimate surfaces, according to the agency.

6

The Economic Effects of the COVID-19 Coronavirus Around the World

As China grapples with the coronavirus, the economic damage is mounting around the world. There are around 70,000 confirmed cases of COVID-19, the new coronavirus that emerged in Wuhan, China, in December and is spreading around the world.

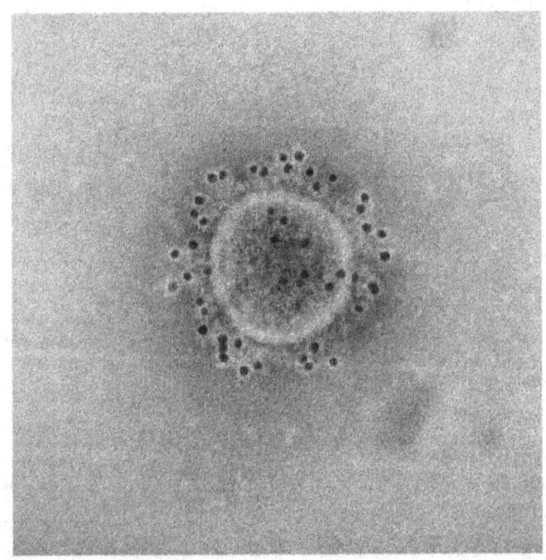

Businesses are dealing with lost revenue and disrupted supply chains due to China's factory shutdowns, tens of millions of people remaining in lockdown in dozens of cities and other countries extending travel restrictions. With many companies and countries depending on the health of China's economy, here are a few ways the outbreak is sending ripples around the world.

Predicted slump

China is the world's second-largest economy and leading trading nation, so economic fallout from coronavirus also threatens global growth.

Economists polled by Reuters between 7-13 February said they expected China's economic growth to slump to 4.5% in the first quarter of 2020, down from 6% in the previous quarter – the slowest pace since the financial crisis.

However, the economists were optimistic China's economy would recover quickly if the virus could be contained.

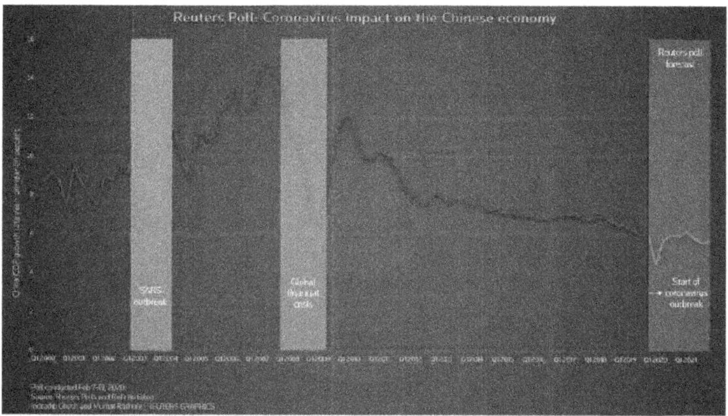

China's economy predicted to grow at its slowest rate since the financial crisis.

Falling oil demand

China is the world's biggest oil importer. With coronavirus hitting manufacturing and travel, the International Energy Agency (IEA) has predicted the first drop in global oil demand in a decade.

"Global oil demand has been hit hard by the novel coronavirus (COVID-19) and the widespread shutdown of China's economy. Demand is now expected to fall by 435,000 barrels year-on-year in the first quarter of 2020, the first quarterly contraction in more than 10 years," the IEA said in its latest monthly report.

Disruption to commerce

The shortage of products and parts from China is affecting companies around the world, as factories delayed opening after the Lunar New Year and workers stayed home to help reduce the spread of the virus.

What is the World Economic Forum doing about epidemics? Apple's manufacturing partner in China, Foxconn, is facing a production delay. Some carmakers including Nissan and Hyundai temporarily closed factories outside China because they couldn't get parts. The pharmaceutical industry is also bracing for disruption to global production. Many trade shows and sporting events in China and across Asia have been cancelled or postponed.

The travel and tourism industries were hit early on by economic disruption from the outbreak.

Global airline revenues are expected to fall by $4-5 billion in the first quarter of 2020 as a result of flight cancellations, according to a report from the UN's International Civil Aviation Organization (ICAO). ICAO also forecasts that Japan could lose $1.29 billion of tourism revenue in the first quarter due to the drop in Chinese travellers while Thailand could lose $1.15 billion.

IMPACT OF COVID-19 ON THE CHINESE AND GLOBAL ECONOMY

The outbreak of the novel coronavirus (COVID-19) is for the time being the most significant black swan of 2020 apart from the increased tensions between the US and Iran which could adversely affect not only the Chinese but the global economy as well.

On 31 December 2019, the World Health Organization (WHO) China Country Office was informed of cases of pneumonia unknown etiology detected in Wuhan City, Hubei Province of China. The Chinese authorities identified a new type of coronavirus, which was isolated on 7 January 2020. On 30 January 2020, WHO issued a Public Health Emergency of International Concern. As of 16 February 2020, WHO reported 51,857 confirmed cases worldwide affecting 25 countries with the epicenter in the south-eastern part of mainland China with 51,174 confirmed cases (with the highest number of cases in Hubei (38839), Guangdong (1316), Zhejiang (1167) and Henan (1231)). The number of deaths reported so far amounts to 1666 in China and 3 abroad. WHO asses the risk of the global pandemic as high and with reference to China as very high. At this stage, we do not fully understand how the 2019-nCoV spreads. This makes containment efforts difficult. WHO officials state clearly that at this stage one cannot predict the direction, duration, scope and scale of the epidemic. This creates an extra dose of uncertainty. Some experts expect the outbreak to last at least until May 2020.

The impact of COVID-19 outbreak on the global economy could be more severe than the impacts of the other major outbreaks in recent history e.g.: SARS (2002-2003), MERS-CoV (2012 -), A/H1N1 (2009-2010) or Ebola (2013-2016). For many reasons - the origin of the COVID-19 should be compared to SARS pandemics which originated from the Chinese Guangdong.

SARS or severe acute respiratory syndrome was a viral respiratory disease of animal origin caused by the SARS coronavirus (SARS-CoV). Between November 2002 and July 2003, an outbreak of SARS in the southern China infected in total 8,098 people (mostly in China), resulting in 774 deaths reported in 17 countries (with a fatality rate of 9.6%), with the majority of cases in mainland China (5,327) and Hong Kong (1,755). No cases of SARS have been reported worldwide since 2004. The Chinese government was criticized for mishandling the outbreak and reacting too slowly (the first case was reported on November 16, 2002, and the WHO was informed only on February 14, 2003). In the case of SARS, it took more than half of the year to contain the spread of the virus.

Considering the lessons from SARS, the Chinese government reacted fast and immediately informed the international bodies (such as the WHO). The measures introduced by China to contain the outbreak at its sources are unprecedented - the quarantine has been levied originally on the city of Wuhan (the source of the outbreak) and later extended to the whole province of Hubei (affecting more than 60 million people). Ahead of the National People's Congress to begin on 5 March 2020 Chinese authorities introduced a two-week quarantine for travelers from other regions of China upon visiting Beijing.

The steps taken so far could have slowed down the spread of the disease to the rest of the world. According to the WHO, a widespread community transmission has not been observed outside of China which is encouraging. The outbreak could be more severe than SARS and could be potentially more disastrous for countries with less efficient health systems.

The impact of SARS on the Chinese economy

Looking from hindsight SARS had a limited impact on the Chinese economy over the long term. However, the short-term impact (quarterly) was detectable. China was the world's 6th largest economy in 2003 experiencing high growth rates over a prolonged period. The SARS outbreak caused China's real GDP growth to slow from 10.5% year over year in the first quarter of 2003 to 8.9% in the second quarter of 2003 and then it accelerated to 10.1% in Q3 and 10.5% in the last quarter of 2003. The overall cost of SARS for China is sometimes estimated as high as 0.5 to 1 percentage points (in the counterfactual scenario).

Expansion in Chinese exports, however, remained steady throughout 2003. The global economy was coming out of a downturn in 2001 to 2002 (real GDP growth rates were 1.74% in 2001, 2.05% in 2002 and 2.88% in 2003) and this fueled demand for Chinese goods allowing the economy to smoothly recover from the outbreak. On the other hand, the yoy growth rates in Chinese imports declined significantly from January to April 2003. Overall, the contribution of trade to Chinese growth, however, remained positive.

Retail sales and industrial production in China was however adversely affected. The decrease in the industrial production growth rates was particularly evident from January to May 2003 prior to recovery.

In comparison to the time of the SARS pandemic, the role of China in the global economy has significantly increased. China is currently the second-largest economy of the world after the US. It is the second-largest importer of manufacturing goods (1.674 trillion USD in 2019) accounting for 9.1% of global imports and the largest exporter (2.524 trillion USD in 2019) responsible for 13.7% of global exports. It is a key country for industrial production and has a key significance for global value chains. China's role globally and in the South Asian region, in particular, is currently much greater than in 2003 and the region's economies are more interlinked.

In comparison to 2002-2003 period, the rates of growth are much more moderate with the real GDP growth rate y/y reported at 6.0% in the third quarter of 2019 and 5.8% forecasted for 2020 (this is still significantly above the world average or the growth rates for the advanced states).

The share of China in global exports was the highest in the case of computers, office, communications, and professional equipment (34.1%), textiles, leather, and apparel (32.8%) as well as glass and non-metallic products (23.8%).

The impact could be thus asymmetrically affecting various GVC to a different extent. For instance, despite the share of China of 5.2% in the global exports of transportation equipment and parts, the outages in the production of key parts already have adversely affected production in the automobile industry globally. Some services sectors could be significantly affected including tourism and transportation (e.g. airline sector).

As the outbreak is mostly concentrated in the Hubei province it is worth to look at the structure of the economy of the affected province.

Hubei province in central China is located at the junction of the Yangtze River Economic Belt from east to west and the Beijing-Guangzhou Railway Economic Belt from north to south. The province is bordered by Shaanxi, Henan, Anhui, Jiangxi, Hunan, and Chongqing Municipality.

The province plays a major role as the largest transportation hub of central China with a significant industrial base and is key to the Central Region Development strategy and the development of the Yangtze River Economic Belt. Hubei's GDP ranks 8th among all provinces in China. Major industries located in the Hubei province include a mixture of traditional and hi-tech sectors such as automobiles, food processing, electronics information, equipment manufacturing, textiles, petrochemical as well as iron & steel.

The impact of COVID-19

The strict restrictions introduced by the Chinese government to control the spread of COVID-19 have so far caused a significant reduction in economic activity in particular to Wuhan and Hubei province. It is worth to note that 26 of 31 Chinese regions have announced extended work stoppage for non-essential enterprises (New Year holidays have been extended; confinement was imposed on millions of residents and travel restrictions within China have been imposed). The impact of the coronavirus will mostly hit China's first-quarter growth. It could extend the second quarter as well if the outbreak lasts longer (till May 2020 if the SARS scenario repeats itself). The overall impact is likely to lower the Chinese real GDP growth rate in 2020 to approx. 5.4% Various economic research teams have already cut their forecasts for 2020 by 0.2 to 0.8 percentage points.

Taking the above into account, policymakers increasingly focus on work resumption in order to stabilize economic growth in 2020. The measures include increased financial support, stabilization of labor market conditions and household consumption as well as expansion in investment spending. Financial & monetary policy support measures embrace intensification of countercyclical monetary policy intervention, provision of lower borrowing costs for affected enterprises, loan rollover or extension for affected enterprises, forbidding lending withdrawal and provisions of tax postponements or tax reductions for affected companies.

The Chinese economy is likely to bounce back after the new outbreak is contained with a rise in the activity in the Q2/Q3 of 2020 due to policy measures described above and the expected increase in consumption spending (with a significant increase in retail sales).

The disturbance to industrial production could be more severe due to a drag caused by the prolonged production shutdowns. These create significant supply outages and disruptions to the internal and external logistics networks and trade flows. It is important to note that the current global manufacturing inventories are generally low. If the situation is prolonged, the adjustments to GVC will be necessary with some production shifting to countries not affected by the outbreak. The impact on global trade flows and shipments could thus be significant and last longer.

The unadjusted PMI index for Chinese manufacturing by IHS Markit readout for January 2020 is below the benchmark value of 50.0 points indicating a contraction. It is worth to note that is less severe than the readout last year.

The most recent trade data are currently available for December 2019, so it is difficult to accurately predict the scale of the effect on Chinese exports and imports. The first estimates showing the scale of the actual downturn will become available only in March. The effect on the trade flows will become more evident only from March onwards (May on in the available data) due to the typical two-to-three-month lead time between purchase and delivery.

The recent webinar by the IHS Maritime & Trade team raised several important issues. The coronavirus couldn't come at a worse time for global shipping. The predicted impact is likely to be much larger than SARS. Given the scale of the economic shock, in the very short to medium-term, shipping demand globally is likely to be severely hit. The expected Chinese demand slowdown is already depressing freight rates, hitting market sentiments hard. Commodity shipping, dry bulk and oil tankers are likely to be worst impacted in the short-term. The impact on container lines could be significant as well.

Implications

The economic impact of the outbreak will depend on its duration and severity. The effect for the global economy will obviously depend as well on its geographic scope. If it is contained to a large extent to China, it will impact the country the hardest. If it starts to spread outside, the impact could be significantly more severe affecting, in particular, the ASEAN countries (Hong Kong, Singapore, etc.) or Japan. The disturbances within global value and logistics chains could accumulate if the containment measures will have to be prolonged. The impact could be the largest on economies most linked to or dependent on China. It is worth to note that several economies are already reporting the adverse impact of the outbreak. These include for instance Singapore (Singapore's Prime Minister Lee Hsien Loong is already referring to a potential recession) or Germany (Germany technically registered zero growth in late 2019, and the prospects for the expected turnaround in early 2020 disappear as China is one of the key export destinations and suppliers to German economy).

ECONOMIC IMPACT OF CORONAVIRUS OUTBREAK DEEPENS

The rising cost of the coronavirus outbreak for business and the world economy is expected to become clearer this week as major firms issue trading updates and China reports the toll on its manufacturing sector.

The latest snapshot of industrial activity in the world's second largest economy, due to be published on Monday, is expected to reveal a plunge in Chinese factory output in February as quarantine efforts to contain the disease disrupt supply chains – with damaging consequences for companies around the world.

China's president Xi Jinping warned at the weekend that the coronavirus would have a "relatively big impact on the economy and society". Adding that it would be short-term and controllable, Xi said the government would step up efforts to cushion the blow. The country has taken a number of measures in recent weeks to prop up its economy.

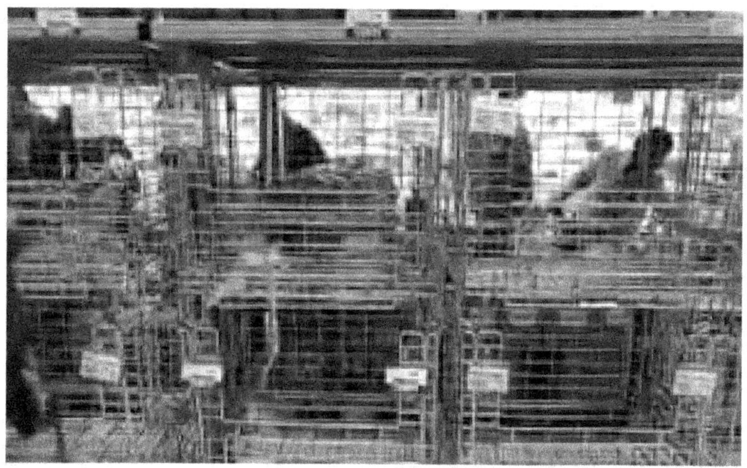

A cluster of coronovirus cases in Lombardy has prompted shoppers to stockpile food, leading to empty shelves such as these at Esselunga in Milan.

The head of the International Monetary Fund, Kristalina Georgieva, said on Sunday that the global lender of last resort was ready to provide additional support, particularly to poorer countries by way of grants and debt relief.

Speaking at a G20 meeting of finance leaders and central bank chiefs, she said the IMF assumed the impact would be relatively minor and shortlived, although she warned that the continued spread of the virus could have dire consequences.

She added: "Global cooperation is essential to the containment of the Covid-19 and its economic impact, particularly if the outbreak turns out to be more persistent and widespread."

Efforts to prevent the spread of the disease were ramped up dramatically over the weekend by Italian authorities, raising the potential to harm eurozone growth at a time when the country's economy is already in contraction.

More than 76,000 people in 27 countries have been infected by the new strain of coronavirus, known as Covid-19, that originated in the Chinese city of Wuhan at the turn of the year. More than 2,200 people have died.

International Airlines Group, the owner of British Airways and Iberia, is scheduled to provide an update on its financial performance for 2019 on Friday that will be closely watched for updates about any potential future impact.

The International Air Transport Association (IATA), the trade body for the global airline industry, warned last week that falling passenger demand would cost the airline industry $29.3bn (£23.7bn) in lost revenues this year, with global air travel expected to fall for the first time in more than a decade.

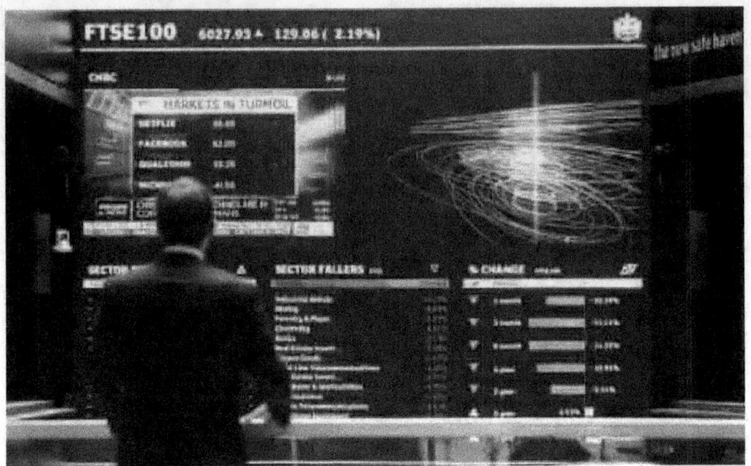

Luxury goods group Hermès will also provide an update to investors on Wednesday. Analysts have warned that transport groups, hospitality chains, airlines, luxury goods makers and retailers will be among those hardest hit by the coronavirus as Chinese consumers stay away from the shops and travellers put off holiday plans.

There are also concerns for global supply chains as Chinese factories remain closed. Jaguar Land Rover warned last week it could run out of car parts at its British factories by next week. The car manufacturer admitted it had been bringing in parts from China to the UK in suitcases.

Apple also sounded the alarm, warning of possible iPhone supply shortages because of the closure of its Chinese factories.

As 2020 begins... ... we're asking readers, like you, to make a new year contribution in support of the Guardian's open, independent journalism. This has been a turbulent decade across the world – protest, populism, mass migration and the escalating climate crisis. The Guardian has been in every corner of the globe, reporting with tenacity, rigour and authority on the most critical events of our lifetimes. At a time when factual information is both scarcer and more essential than ever, we believe that each of us deserves access to accurate reporting with integrity at its heart.

You've read more than 20 articles in the last four months. More people than ever before are reading and supporting our journalism, in more than 180 countries around the world. And this is only possible because we made a different choice: to keep our reporting open for all, regardless of where they live or what they can afford to pay.

We have upheld our editorial independence in the face of the disintegration of traditional media – with social platforms giving rise to misinformation, the seemingly unstoppable rise of big tech and independent voices being squashed by commercial ownership. The Guardian's independence means we can set our own agenda and voice our own opinions. Our journalism is free from commercial and political bias – never influenced by billionaire owners or shareholders. This makes us different. It means we can challenge the powerful without fear and give a voice to those less heard.

None of this would have been attainable without our readers' generosity – your financial support has meant we can keep investigating, disentangling and interrogating. It has protected our independence, which has never been so critical. We are so grateful.

JAPAN AND AUSTRALIA ECONOMIES ALREADY FEELING IMPACT FROM COVID-19

Key gauges for manufacturing in Australia and Japan have fallen while early export orders for South Korea show a slump in Chinese demand.

The warning signs come as finance chiefs from the Group of 20 (G20), the world's 20 biggest economies, meet this weekend in Riyadh for the first time since the virus was first detected in humans.

How to cope with the economic fallout from the disease will dominate those discussions, Bank of Japan Gov. Haruhiko Kuroda said in Tokyo ahead of his departure for the talks.

Manufacturing activity in Japan plunged amid recession risks in the world's third largest economy. The Jibun Bank Japan Manufacturing Purchasing Managers' Index registered 47.6 for the sharpest deterioration in conditions in more than seven years.

The epidemic has prompted economists to forecast recession in Japan's economy, which was already reeling from an October sales tax hike and a typhoon.

In Australia a gauge of manufacturing activity fell further into negative territory as effects of the virus have spread, along with a hit from massive bush fires.

The CBA Flash Composite PMI fell to 48.3 in February from 50.2, the steepest rate of reduction since the series began in May 2016.

While early South Korea trade figures for February indicated some improvement, an increased number of working days from a year earlier glossed over the impact the virus is already having.

Exports during the first 20 days of the month rose 12 percent from a year earlier. Shipments to China, South Korea's biggest trade partner, fell 3.7 percent during the first 20 days. The early reading is typically held up as a bellwether for global trade given South Korea's central role as a manufacturer and exporter of electronics, ships and automobiles.

Economists warn the fallout of COVID-19 is only just beginning.

"The global economy and financial markets have not seen the full impact of the coronavirus outbreak yet," Citigroup economists led by Catherine Mann wrote in a note titled "Waiting for the Global Impact" that warned of a "dramatic" first quarter slowdown in China.

Slumping activity will add to pressure on governments and central banks to respond with more support for their economies, while also raising doubts about their capacity to do so.

Central banks in Asia have already stepped up action, with Indonesia, the Philippines and Thailand cutting rates recently, and others like Singapore planning significant fiscal stimulus. China has lowered a range of policy rates this month. Speculation is rising that the Bank of Korea could also deliver a cut next week.

Still, global debt is at record levels and interest rates in the world's biggest economies are already at historic lows.

"If growth continues to slide, a key question for the G20 will be whether its members can coordinate a response," according to Bloomberg Economics' Tom Orlik.

"Against a backdrop of resurgent nationalism, fractious trade disputes, and limited policy space, common purpose might be difficult to achieve, that's another reason to be pessimistic on the outlook," he wrote.

ONCE WIDELY CRITICIZED, THE WUHAN QUARANTINE BOUGHT THE WORLD TIME TO PREPARE FOR COVID-19

When the Chinese government blocked most travel into and out of the city at the center of the Covid-19 outbreak in late January, many public health experts took to social media and op-ed pages to decry the measure as not only draconian and a violation of individual rights but also as ineffective: This largest quarantine in history — the city, Wuhan, has a population of 11 million, and the lockdown has been expanded — would have little effect on the course of the epidemic, they argued.

As the U.S. and other countries imposed travel restrictions, even the World Health Organization questioned whether they were a good idea. But early evidence is causing some disease fighters to reconsider.

The last few days have seen a perceptible flattening in growth of Covid-19 cases in China, raising hopes that the epidemic has peaked. (Though there are doubts about the accuracy of China's count.) That supports the emerging consensus on the

Wuhan quarantine in particular: that, at minimum, it bought China and the world time to prepare. Crucially, the time lag allowed public health agencies to devise and distribute a diagnostic test that hospitals can use to identify patients ill with the novel coronavirus.

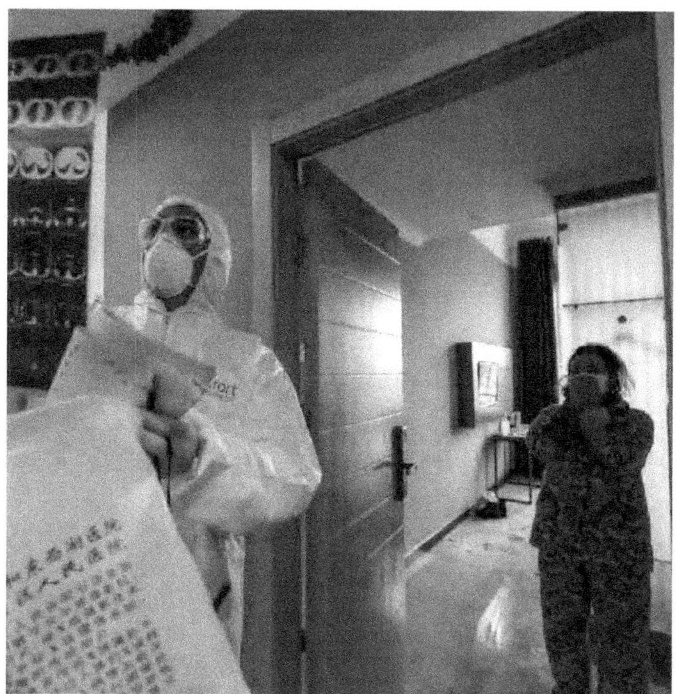

A doctor looks at a lung CT scan at a hospital in the quarantine zone in Wuhan, China

"Measures on movement restriction have delayed the dissemination of the outbreak two or three days within China and a few weeks outside China," Sylvie Briand, director of Infectious Hazard Management at the WHO, told reporters this week. "Those measures, if well implemented, could have an impact on the propagation of the outbreak."

Scientists are still gathering data on the effect of travel restrictions and the historic quarantine — and, in particular, whether they reduced total cases and deaths or just postponed many of them without lowering the eventual cumulative toll. The answer will have broad consequences for future outbreaks, perhaps putting large-scale quarantines back on the list of health officials' epidemic countermeasures, including in countries that value individual liberties more than China does.

"We should do what we can to understand their effectiveness, because [quarantines and travel restrictions] may be considered again in this epidemic and in future epidemics," said preparedness expert Tom Inglesby, director of the Center for Health

Security of the Johns Hopkins Bloomberg School of Public Health. "It's important to know not only if they worked in some way but also to gauge if they did harm."

There have, in fact, been numerous, and in some cases fatal, unintended knock-on effects of the quarantine, as critics warned. People were unable to reach sick, elderly parents in Wuhan, let alone take them out of the city for treatment of heart disease, cancer, diabetes, and other illnesses. This week, UNAIDS announced that one-third of people in China who are living with HIV reported that because of lockdowns and travel restrictions they were at risk of running out of their HIV medications within days. And China's economy has slowed to a crawl.

The impact of the movement restrictions extends beyond Wuhan, to other areas in China as well as other countries getting a trickle of cases early this month rather than the flood they likely would have if Wuhan residents and visitors had been able to leave the city. As a result, they have been able to deploy countermeasures with deliberation and not in a rushed panic.

The quarantine "let countries field the fly balls coming at them one by one by one and not drop them," said David Fisman of the University of Toronto, a leading epidemic modeler. "The fact that Wuhan got sealed off made the numbers something other countries could handle. They've been able to figure out things like how to identify cases and what to do with them. I think that made a huge difference."

If thousands of infected people had traveled from Wuhan starting in late January, Fisman said, "every place new cases landed would have had the potential to be another Wuhan," whose Hubei province is approaching 2,000 deaths.

Instead, health care systems in countries that have had cases (1,073 and counting outside China, according to WHO) had time to prepare, said Alexandra Phelan of Georgetown University's Center for Global Health Science and Security: "Delays can be a really useful tool, and maybe one of the only tools you have, to implement screening and training for health care workers, and essentially get your house in order."

Hospitals could have used the time to give their staffs refresher courses in infection control and practice using respiratory gear, said Inglesby (though it's not clear how many in which countries did so). Agencies such as the U.S. Centers for Disease Control and Prevention had time to update and disseminate technical information, including the use of diagnostic kits.

"The ability to test for the virus has been distributed pretty widely," including by the CDC to U.S. states and cities, Inglesby said. Testing capacity grew outside the U.S., too, he said: "Certainly more countries can test for the virus now than three weeks ago," when without the Wuhan quarantine they might have faced a flood of cases, both suspected and real.

With the breathing room the quarantine provided, China has been able to plan or begin about 120 clinical trials of potential Covid-19 treatments, Inglesby added: "There has been time to acquire data on what medications might work," including those currently in use for other diseases and therefore relatively available.

U.S. travel restrictions (barring most foreign nationals who have been in China recently from entering, requiring Americans returning from China to be quarantined or self-isolate) were, like the Wuhan quarantine, "really meant to slow down the spread" of the coronavirus, Health and Human Services Secretary Alex Azar, told reporters this month. "It's not meant to hermetically seal the United States from the virus, but rather to allow us to focus our resources," including by setting up the quarantine centers. "It's about slowing spread."

"I think most health officials agree that at best [quarantine or travel restriction] delays and ... kind of pauses things," Anthony Fauci, director of the National Institute of Allergy and Infectious Diseases, told reporters. "What we needed was a delay to essentially prepare better."

Experts are divided, however, on whether the Wuhan quarantine not only resulted in what the WHO's Briand called "postponing the peak" of the epidemic — the time when the number of new cases tops out — but also in reducing the total number of cases and deaths.

"I haven't seen anything that says the overall number of people infected in the world will be less" than without the Wuhan quarantine, Inglesby said.

The reason for pessimism is that although the quarantine reduced the rate of transmission and therefore the number of cases in any given time period, normal commercial activity and travel in China "has to resume at some point, so it's hard to argue that the disease wouldn't resume its trajectory," Inglesby said. "No one has put forth the case that what China has done will eliminate this virus from Earth." Sustained transmission, however, might look more like bad colds (as other coronaviruses cause) than like severe seasonal flu.

Experts who take a more sanguine view believe that slowing the spread and buying time for countermeasures did have a permanent effect on the epidemic, not only postponing what would have been today's cases into next week but preventing some of those cases forever. If so, then the eventual toll would be less than without the Wuhan quarantine.

That and other control measures changed how many cases each infected person causes "big time," Fisman said. The lower this "reproductive number," the lower the total case count. The Wuhan quarantine, he said, "reduced the likelihood of people in Wuhan coming into contact with people not in Wuhan. The rate of transmission is now pretty flat. This is coming under control in other cities [outside Hubei] in China."

Fisman's and other mathematical models of the epidemic's trajectory, however, are undermined by the fact that key numbers in the equations describing disease transmission (a "model" is essentially a group of equations solved by computers) are uncertain.

For instance, the time between when one infected person becomes ill and when someone he infects does was thought to be five to seven days. But an analysis led by Hiroshi Nishiura of Japan's Hokkaido University suggests this "serial interval" is only four days.

That could be bad news because half the people who get sick do so less than four days after exposure to the virus that causes Covid-19. "A substantial proportion" of transmission may therefore occur before people show symptoms, Nishiura and his colleagues warned. "Pre-symptomatic transmission … may even occur more frequently than symptomatic transmission," confounding control measures: If people can spread disease before they're sick, then isolating only sick people won't stop transmission.

In fact, physicians in China reported this week in the New England Journal of Medicine that a symptom-free individual had just as much virus (according to nose and throat swabs) as patients with symptoms — all set to be sneezed or coughed onto other people.

Although diseases that can be spread by people who aren't sick are harder to control, there are hints that the worst of the Covid-19 outbreak in China is nevertheless past. Like several other models, three by researchers at Georgia State University School of Public Health projecting Covid-19 cases suggest that the outbreak is losing steam. Total cases in China outside Hubei should stay below 15,000 through the end of February, with little increase after that, the models say. (Projections for Hubei got scrambled when China changed the case definition for Covid-19, producing a sharp one-time uptick in case totals last week.)

As of Thursday, there were 12,644 Covid-19 cases in China outside Hubei.

"For all other provinces, the models are on track," said mathematical epidemiologist Gerardo Chowell of Georgia State. "The containment strategies implemented in China are successfully reducing transmission," he and his colleagues wrote in a paper published last week in Infectious Disease Modeling. "The epidemic growth has slowed."

Chowell inclines toward optimism, he said: "I think that we'll control this," especially if the Covid-19 virus (like influenza and other viruses) doesn't survive or spread as well in warm, humid conditions.

Barring secondary outbreaks (as happened with SARS, a coronavirus that spread around the globe in 2003), Chowell said, the Covid-19 epidemic in China might be over in three weeks. This pathogen might join the other four coronaviruses that give millions of people colds and, in some cases, pneumonia every year. If it falls well short of an uncontrollable pandemic, quarantines and other measures widely viewed as ineffective and even counterproductive could well join the bag of tools used in future viral outbreaks.

CORONAVIRUS IS DEVASTATING CHINESE TOURISM

Countries have closed off their borders with China, airlines have slashed flights, and hotels have seen a big drop-off in bookings.

Last month, on January 19, Myanmar's state-run newspaper left no question as to what was the biggest story of the day. The paper carried page after page of dry reports documenting the movements and meetings of visiting Chinese President Xi Jinping. Inside were photos of Xi and Myanmar's leader, Aung San Suu Kyi, sitting in gilded chairs behind a table draped in red, yellow, and green fabric, the colors of Myanmar's flag. A parade of officials had taken turns posing in front of them, clutching red folios that each contained one of the dozens of freshly signed agreements between the two countries. The visit marked the start of the "Myanmar-China Bilateral Cultural and Tourism Year."

Buried inside the same edition of the paper was a single article, plucked from the AFP newswire, detailing alarm by medical experts in London over the spread of a "mysterious SARS-like virus in China" and warning that the scale of the outbreak was "likely far bigger than officially reported." Of the two stories, this is the one proving to be more important to Myanmar, Southeast Asia, and the world.

The illness, now officially labeled COVID-19, has raced across the globe, infecting tens of thousands of people and killing more than 2,000, predominantly in China. Countries have closed their borders to Chinese travelers; airlines have slashed flights and limited routes. Points of transit across Asia—train stations, bus depots, airports— have seen traffic plummet, and some are nearly deserted. Leaders in Beijing are undertaking a sprawling lockdown and quarantine on a scale that is difficult to comprehend. The impact on the global economy is still yet to be fully understood.

Powered by a middle class expanding in both wealth and size, the Chinese tourism market has seen staggering growth over the past two decades. Travel departures from China, according to the United Nations World Tourism Organization, increased from

4.5 million in 2000 to 150 million in 2018. These travelers have become their own economic force, spending $277 billion, and many countries have rushed to embrace them. Yet if Western countries have experienced the growing number of Chinese tourists as simply a boon for the economy, around Asia the influx of visitors has been even more transformative. All of the top 10 destinations for Chinese visitors last year were in Asia, according to the China Outbound Tourism Research Institute, and the results are evident to any traveler in the region: signs at travel hubs that include directions in Chinese, tourism staff who speak at least a smattering of the language, shops that accept mobile payments from Chinese apps. (At the same time, stories of Chinese tourists behaving badly and complaints of "zero dollar" tourism, whereby locals see little money from inbound visitors, have also risen.)

But now, as COVID-19 sharply curtails travel across the region, analysts and governments of countries that have become heavily reliant on Chinese visitors—some overly so—are dampening their forecasts. More than 40,000 hotel bookings on the Indonesian island of Bali have been canceled, according to officials there, and the outbreak could shave up to 0.3 percentage points off the country's GDP growth. Billions of dollars in tourism spending are projected to be lost by Vietnam. Tourists from China are the largest group of visitors to Thailand, but the government expects the annual number of Chinese travelers to fall by at least 2 million. A hotel manager in the Thai city of Chiang Mai told me the situation was a "total mess," as travel agents and hotels scrambled to reschedule and collect payments from canceled tour groups. Immigration figures for the city's airport show a near-total collapse in the number of arrivals from China starting in late January. Casinos in Macau, the world's gambling capital, normally teeming with players from the mainland, are shuttered. Lisa Wan, a professor at Chinese University of Hong Kong Business School, was blunt in her assessment: "The global tourism industry is expected to suffer massively during the outbreak," she told me.*

Few places illustrate this economic relationship with China—capitalizing on an incredible growth in tourism and trade, thereby building a dependence that creates a vulnerability—like Myanmar. The country's tourism sector has rapidly expanded since the government undertook political and economic reforms in 2011, but in 2018, arrivals from the United States and Europe dropped 50 percent, in part because of a military campaign carried out near Myanmar's western border. Looking to rebound, the government aggressively courted the Asian market, rolling out visa exemptions and new flight connections to numerous Chinese cities, including Chongqing, Haikou, and Wuhan, the center of the latest virus outbreak—the international airport in Mandalay now almost exclusively services China. Arrivals from there rose from 20 percent of the overall figure in 2018 to 38 percent in 2019, according to the World

Bank. May Myat Mon Win, a vice chair of the Myanmar Tourism Federation, told me that tour organizers from China had in recent years taken to booking all the rooms in some budget hotels for every night of the year, sometimes for two years at a time—unlike tourists from elsewhere, Chinese visitors traveled year-round.

Thant Zin Tun, a hotel owner with properties across Myanmar managed by international brands, began to cater to the new guests, hiring Chinese speakers and expanding menu options. The first offerings of the day needed adapting, for example, because Chinese tourists "don't really fancy the European, Western breakfast," he said he had learned. But since the COVID-19 outbreak, he said he had seen an 85 percent drop in business at his hotels in Mandalay and Bagan, an area covered with ancient temples, both places where Chinese tourists have flocked to in recent years.

And at Yangon's Bogyoke Market on a recent Saturday, tourists, particularly those from China, were largely missing. Saleswomen with no customers to entertain chatted among themselves and tapped on their phones behind glass cases displaying bracelets, pendants, and jade ornaments in shades varying from milky white to deep emerald.

Sitting under one of the market's covered walkways, Zin Min Tun, who has run half a dozen pearl and gem shops since 1996, estimated that the number of Chinese tourists over the previous month had dropped roughly 70 percent compared with last year.

His fingers wrapped in thick ruby and agate rings, Zin Min Tun said Chinese tourists were the biggest buyers of jade, mined in Myanmar's north, and the country's pearls, which have a champagne-colored sheen. "The whole world depends on China," he said. "Now they have money; they can spend around the world, not just Myanmar."

The concerns Thant Zin Tun and other spoke of were reflected by analysts at Fitch Solutions, who last week said they were lowering their forecast for Myanmar's GDP growth, noting that tourism would be "subdued over the coming months due to lower Chinese visitors from China's ban on travel agent bookings, and also risk aversion from tourists of other nationalities due to Myanmar's weak patient tracking capability." (Upon my flight's arrival into Yangon airport, workers in hazmat suits armed with thermometers entered the plane and took our temperatures.)

While Thant Zin Tun bemoaned the lost business, May Myat Mon Win, the tourism federation vice chair, was quick to remind me that Myanmar was hardly the only country feeling the downturn and that others were even more reliant on Chinese visitors. "China is a giant, the dragon," she told me. "If the dragon is hit harder than this, I think there is going to be more consequences for the global economy and, of course, tourism."

One such area is Macau, the former Portuguese colony, which welcomed nearly 28 million visitors from mainland China last year, about 70 percent of all arrivals. (Macau is now a special administrative region that is part of China but, like Hong Kong, has a separate legal system, judiciary, and immigration regime.)

Though Macau's economy is almost wholly dependent on gaming, after a string of confirmed COVID-19 cases, the government forced all 41 casinos to halt operations for a 15-day period starting on February 5. Numerous hotels have temporarily shuttered as a result, and residents are largely abiding by the government's recommendation to stay home. The gondolas used to ferry tourists through the artificial canals at the Venetian Hotel sat empty on the mouthwash-blue water, opera music echoing off the faux-Italian-building fronts. One security guard standing in front of a stopped escalator at the Parisian Hotel said that without any visitors, things had gotten "very boring." A sales attendant in a luxury boutique busied himself by styling a mannequin, removing and replacing a pair of sunglasses and tweaking a bucket hat before settling on a final look, then starting again.

CORONAVIRUS IS STARTING TO HIT BIG TECH'S BOTTOM LINE

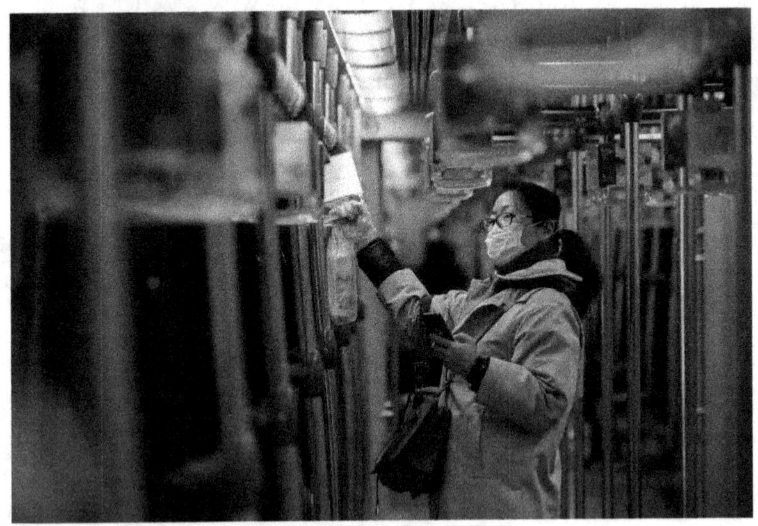

The Covid-19 coronavirus disease has started to impact the businesses of major tech companies like Apple.

The outbreak of the Covid-19 coronavirus disease has taken the lives of over 2,100 people — with all but 11 of those deaths in China — and infected over 75,000 as of February 20. As the world scrambles to contain the public health crisis, global businesses are starting to take a hit, particularly in the technology sector.

China — which is the second-largest economy in the world — has all but halted its production of consumer goods like phones, clothing, and automobiles for the past several weeks. The country has taken on unprecedented "wartime" measures to control the virus's spread, such as placing severe restrictions of some 780 million people and instituting mass quarantines in major cities.

The Wall Street Journal reports that the lockdown on Chinese manufacturing has caused global markets to "shudder" and is casting an "ever-widening shadow" on the economy at large. That's particularly relevant in the tech industry, which depends on Chinese labor to build everything from computer chips to cellphone parts. In recent days, China has started reopening its factories (despite public health concerns) in an effort to restart its economy, but manufacturing sites are still running at a far lower capacity than usual.

It's still too early to measure the full financial impact of the virus on the tech industry, but the early signs don't look good. Apple — the world's most valuable tech company — said it is reducing its revenue targets this quarter in a rare company advisory released on Monday. Tesla said last week that "health epidemics" are a risk to its business. Amazon, whose e-commerce business relies on the flow of goods between China, the US, and other countries, has not released any similar warnings but is stockpiling supplier items from China to protect against future disruptions due to the virus. And Chinese companies themselves are feeling the hit, with tech giant Alibaba calling the outbreak a "black swan" event (as in, unpredictable) on a recent earnings call.

Social media companies — which are trying to keep up with a slew of misinformation about the virus's origins and spread — are still financially less impacted than companies like Apple since their main line of business isn't selling physical goods. But even Facebook has been affected, setting reduced production goals for its Oculus Quest virtual reality headsets in part due to a slowdown in Chinese manufacturing because of the virus.

And virtually all the major tech companies — Apple, Google, Facebook, Amazon, and Microsoft — have restricted employee travel to China, either banning or limiting it only to matters of critical importance. They're also asking workers returning from China to work from home for up to two weeks.

In some cases, tech professionals in the US are so concerned about the virus that they're taking other precautions, such as wearing breathing masks and eliminating handshakes in business meetings, as Recode previously reported. For now, there are only four confirmed cases in the San Francisco Bay Area, but some feel these preventative measures are important given the high volume of travel between China and Silicon Valley — and concerns that the virus could quickly grow out of control given how it has spread in Asia.

Overall, the economic and social impact the coronavirus is having on the tech industry puts into stark relief the close connection between Silicon Valley and China, not just for manufacturing but for supplying a workforce of highly skilled engineers, investor funds, and academic collaboration.

Outside the workplace, tech companies are pulling out of major global conferences or canceling them altogether. As Recode reported last week, Facebook canceled a 5,000-person global marketing conference in San Francisco. And the world's largest phone trade show, Mobile World Congress, was canceled after major tech companies like Amazon pulled out over coronavirus concerns.

Here are more specifics on some of the main ways we are seeing coronavirus impact the global economy, particularly in the tech industry.

Supply chain disruption

Virtually every major US tech company that builds physical products — like cellphones, computers, or video game consoles — relies on a vast Chinese workforce to manufacture products for cheaper than could be done in the US.

In the past few weeks, though, that supply chain, which includes everything from raw parts to finished products, has been fundamentally disrupted.

Factories in China have been shut down. Hundreds of millions of migrant workers who were visiting family in cities outside the main manufacturing hubs for Chinese New Year were quarantined. Some are beginning to return to work, but reports indicate that as of earlier this week, over two-thirds remain stuck. Roads have been blocked, trains halted, and flights canceled.

In its advisory, Apple said Monday that "worldwide iPhone supply will be temporarily constrained" because its manufacturing sites in China are "experiencing a slower return to normal conditions" than anticipated as manufacturing sites in the region slowly reopen.

The New York Times reports that even though some factories are starting up again, they are still "operating well below capacity." And there are serious public health concerns about whether reopening the factories is the right decision at all, considering the virus continues to spread in China and elsewhere.

Companies are increasingly talking about the threat of the virus in public business announcements. A MarketWatch report found that out of the S&P 500 companies' recent earnings calls between January 1 and February 13, 38 percent of transcripts included the term "coronavirus" at least once.

Another major tech company with its supply chain impacted by the virus is

Amazon. It's estimated that over 40 percent of Amazon sellers are based in China, which means that a large chunk of the products people buy comes from the country. In addition to that, a large portion of US-based sellers source their products from China.

According to a recent Business Insider report, Amazon reached out last week to a number of suppliers for products sold in the US but made in China and encouraged them "to stockpile on certain products shipped from China, in anticipation of potential supply chain slowdowns caused by the coronavirus outbreak in the region," according to the outlet.

In response to a question about this practice, Amazon sent Recode the following statement: "Out of an abundance of caution, we are working with suppliers to secure additional inventory to ensure we maintain our selection for customers."

Facebook also said the manufacturing of its Oculus Quest headsets is impacted by the outbreak.

"Oculus Quest has been selling out in some regions due to high demand," Facebook spokesperson Anthony Harrison wrote in a statement to Recode.

"That said, like other companies, we're expecting some additional impact to our hardware production due to the coronavirus. We're taking precautions to ensure the safety of our employees, manufacturing partners and customers, and are monitoring the situation closely. We are working to restore availability as soon as possible."

Chinese demand

Another way the coronavirus outbreak is impacting business is by reducing Chinese consumers' demand for consumer electronics.

China is the United States' third-largest and most rapidly growing market for exports, which means that US companies are increasingly setting revenue goals that rely on Chinese residents buying their products.

Apple in particular made a whopping $52 billion in sales in the last fiscal year by selling its products (mostly iPhones) in the country. With the recent easing of tensions in the US-China trade war, analysts were anticipating that number to grow at a faster rate than it had in previous months.

But now, because of the coronavirus, that could all change. Apple temporarily closed some of its more than 40 stores in the country and is currently still operating some under limited hours.

The company said on an earnings call that there has been "very low customer traffic" in its stores.

CHINA'S TOURISM, AUTOMOTIVE INDUSTRIES SINK AMID COVID-19 OUTBREAK

China's extraordinary economic growth over the past four decades transformed the country into the world's second-biggest economy.

The key to this growth is global trade. China is not only the largest trading partner in the world, but it is also central to a myriad of supply chains. From raw materials to components used in electronics, Chinese companies work hard to provide Western brands with inexpensive building blocks for their next expensive product, be it a car, a smartphone or some other widget. (Apple AAPL, -2.26% said Feb. 17 it won't meet its quarterly financial guidance. It generates about 15% of its revenue from China, and many of its products are manufactured there.)

The Wuhan coronavirus (now officially named COVID-19) has thrown a wrench into this well-oiled machine, and the Chinese economy could grind to a halt, dragging down global growth with it.

The first area to suffer is tourism. In the third quarter, 173 million Chinese tourists went abroad. Some experts say the number of travelers has already fallen by 55% compared with 2019's Lunar New Year (Feb. 5). Chinese tourists are big spenders, so the travel ban will hurt the bottom lines of their favorite tourist destinations — Cambodia, Thailand and Hong Kong. In 2017, the World Tourism Organization said China was the largest contributor to the global outbound tourism market, spending almost $258 billion in that year alone.

Automotive industry

Many companies all over the world do business with China, and the disruption in supply chains will result in unavoidable delays in their endeavors to introduce new products to the market. This is especially true for the automotive industry because Hubei province, where the outbreak first occurred, is a big center of automotive supply manufacturers.

According to DHL's supply chain risk assessment service, half of all manufacturing in Wuhan is related to the automotive industry. "The regional lockdown has already severely impeded logistics operations that rely on access to highways to carry goods into and out of the region, while severe delays should also be expected on inbound and outbound air cargo shipments," the DHL report said.

It is estimated that the disruption and delays now in place due to countermeasures to the deadly virus will slash production by about 15% in the first quarter. This will affect Toyota TM, -0.05%, Volkswagen VOW, -1.35% and General Motors GM, -1.81%, among other car companies.

That estimate doesn't take into account the possibility of plants remaining closed into mid-March. If that happens, the situation becomes more dire — lost production of more than 1.7 million units for the first quarter, or about a 32.3% drop from IHS Markit's initial expectations before the crisis began.

COVID-19 vs SARS

Many are tempted to compare COVID-19 to the SARS outbreak, but Neil Shearing, group chief economist at Capital Economics, begs to differ: "While it's tempting to draw comparisons to the SARS epidemic in 2003, China's economy is now much larger and more closely integrated into global supply chains. An economic shock in China is now more likely to spread to the rest of the world. ... The potential for the [Wuhan] virus to trigger a significant market correction is much greater now than it was back then [during the SARS outbreak]."

Work on vaccines

But things don't necessarily need to be that grim. What experts do agree on is that, even if global GDP suffers further as a result of the virus' impact, the global economy will rebound after it's under control. This, however, should be considered in light of the latest claims by the World Health Organization's director-general, Tedros Adhanom Ghebreyesus, who estimated that the development of the vaccine for COVID-19 will take about 18 months. Pharmaceutical company GlaxoSmithKline GSK, +0.75% came out with a time frame of as little as 12 months, and at least a dozen other companies are working on a solution to the COVID-19 outbreak.

Companies will adapt

What's more likely to happen: International supply-demand mechanisms will adapt and find alternative routes of fulfillment, eliminating China as a partner where necessary, even if it means doing business at more unfavorable prices. After the crisis is averted, we can expect the old trade routes to re-emerge and business with China to continue as usual.

The only question now is how long it will take to eliminate the viral threat, and at what cost will global companies be able to wean themselves off Chinese exports, cover their losses and establish similar partnerships with businesses outside China.

WORLD ECONOMY WILL BE FACING CHINA'S CORONAVIRUS FOR A LONG TIME

Everywhere we look we see the headlines and commentators talking about the coronavirus and its impact on tourism, trade and investment between China and the

West — and China and the U.S., in particular. However, there are far-reaching effects that have not been contemplated fully beyond the intuitive assessment.

Things move slowly. China has long been known as a country with patience, which in business language translates to longer lead times in the transactional arena, sometimes exhaustive negotiations, and relationships are built over time. Many of these relationships are created in the environment of trade shows, conferences, information exchange platforms, and trade delegations. China has finely tuned this method of cross-border introductions and it is a continuous process.

Combined with this is the growth of the multinational business presence in China. Major retailers, manufacturers, pharmaceuticals, biotech, automotive and other sectors are firmly planted in China with technology and personnel. Now, with the essentially closed border with China, the rest of the world waits and watches. To the business community, this is unsettling, to say the least, because there is no accurate predictor of when a vaccine may be found or when the world threat eradicated. Even when those pronouncements are ultimately made by Beijing there is the inherent distrust of information disseminated by the Chinese government.

So what does all of this mean for cross-border business in the short and long term?

An aerial view reveals that the movement of people and technology and deal closure have simply come to a halt. When the Chinese government, or other governments, or the WHO pronounce that it is safe to travel to China again, that will not be the end of it. There has been a worldwide reaction to the scare. The tradeshow and related cancellations have occurred not only in China but throughout Asia and into Europe. Therefore, a wide swath of activities are upended across all business sectors.

As of this writing, there have been more than 45,000 cases of Covid-19 and over 1,100 deaths. Businesses from cruise ships to luxury brands and air travel, as well as global markets like oil, have all been hit. There can be no question that it will be a slow and painful process moving back to normalcy. Professional offices remain closed indefinitely, and 90% of businesses are closed or at dramatically reduced hours. Theaters, factories and others where people congregate are closed.

The headlines today paint Wuhan as a pariah city, in a wartime battle and in lockdown. The Chinese Chernobyl. These characterizations will not be easily shed.

We are all familiar with the recent comparisons of coronavirus with SARS, but there is no real comparison. SARS was perceived as essentially a Hong Kong-centric event and everyone wondered if that would be the death of the HK economy, coming a few years after the handover. Moreover, social media and its impact on global interaction were just launching, and China's interaction with the world economy was in its infancy.

Transparency will be the key to short term confidence which will lead to a long-term recovery. This is despite short-term pain and embarrassment. All governments can learn a lesson from this, but Beijing has yet to learn it. It may very well be that Wuhan, as ground zero for the Coronavirus, never recovers. The headlines today paint Wuhan as a pariah city, in a wartime battle and in lockdown. The Chinese Chernobyl. These characterizations will not be easily shed. Wuhan, as the capital of Hubei province, has positioned itself as a foreign investment hub and has developed trade, manufacturing and export and development zones to highlight its growth and position within China. Companies will have to assess whether or not their investments should remain in Wuhan or be moved.

Considering China's impact on the world economy, China will not be off limits to future investment forever. Instead, there will be wariness and unbridled caution for the foreseeable future. Businesses will seek alternatives to avoid commercial and liability issues.

In the best case, returning to normal is not a reasonable expectation in the short term. In the long term, China must take all steps necessary to demonstrate its commitment to transparency regarding all factors relating to the virus. In today's economy, there are many alternatives for trade and investment and China must recognize that its global trade partners need regular and repeated reassurances. Additionally, China will need to inject substantial financial incentives into the economy to balance against commercial and optical risks.

In the best of circumstances, this process will take six to nine months to see the way forward to a stable and commercially feasible reintroduction of business, confidence and renewed investment. This will require unrelenting adjustments as events require. There is no single action or vaccine that will erase the impact of the coronavirus. A group of actions are needed to restore the zeal and excitement for consumer, business, investment and tourism.

Anything less will create a lingering atmosphere of caution and distrust.

7

Coronavirus: New 'Black Swan' of Global Economy

With the impact of trade wars, Brexit and various geopolitical issues, the global economy has been going through a hard time and the possibilities of recession and economic slowdown are on the global agenda. One of the concerns is the fear of a "Black Swan" scenario coming true, further deteriorating the global economy, which has already been on fragile ground for some time. The recent outbreak of the novel coronavirus that emerged in Wuhan, China brought forward the possibility of such a scenario, increasing concerns about the global economy.

Impacts of such outbreaks are hastily interpreted primarily through their impact on exchanges. I believe this to be a faulty choice. Financial markets strongly react to the flow of information about these kinds of unexpected events. An increase in the death toll might suddenly result in a 10% loss of value in stock markets. On the other hand, even a shred of good news could be regarded as an opportunity to buy. Because we are talking about China, which is considered the "factory of the world," it would be wise to assess the impacts through supply chains, foreign trade and real sector channels.

Despite this, thanks to economic stimulus packages by the Chinese government, an increase in export performance and delayed demand being activated in markets later in the year, the Chinese economy succeeded in closing 2003 with a 10% growth rate. It is estimated that global economic growth lost 0.1 percentage point of real GDP due to SARS.

The impacts of the new coronavirus, also called the "Wuhan virus," could be felt more deeply than that of SARS. The Chinese economy compensated for shrinking domestic demand in the second quarter of 2003 by exporting more goods and services. Consequently, export rates of China increased by 35% in 2003. The fact that China became a member of the World Trade Organization in 2001 also had a great role to play in this impressive export performance.

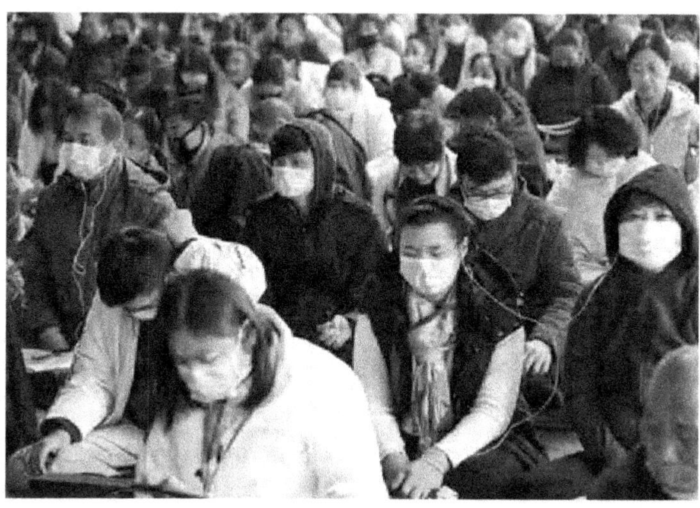

However, China no longer has the same radius of action that would enable it to increase its exports in such significant numbers. In recent years, China has gone through a transformation from an export-based growth model to a model dependent on domestic demand. The share of domestic demand in the growth composition is much heavier now than it was in the past.

In comparison with 2003, China's foreign trade is five times bigger today, the number of tourists sent abroad is six times more and its share from the global economy has also increased fourfold. It would not be a surprise if developments in China impact the global economy more deeply than it would 17 years ago.

The case of SARS happened at a time when risks in the global economy were lower, the desire for investments were higher and trading volume was in a tendency to further increase. But now, along with uncertainties and higher risks, we are going through an era in which global growth and trading volumes hardly move forward due to trade wars. The deterioration of expectations on the global economy might render the impacts of the virus a tad stronger.

How much will these factors increase the negative impact of the Wuhan virus on the economy compared to that of SARS? With reference to the scenario in which the coronavirus outbreak would be under control by April, Shang-Jin Wei from Columbia University made a very optimistic prediction that the impact of the virus on Chinese economic growth would be limited to only 0.1 percentage point. International finance organizations predict that the Chinese economy will experience a loss of growth by 0.5 percentage point on average. There are also grave pessimists who predict that the Chinese economy will face a loss of growth of more than 1 percentage point. Predictions about the overall global economic growth loss due to the virus range between 0.02 to 0.03 percentage point.

Which countries will be affected, and how much?

Based on the present data, it would be wiser to predict the situation in reference to the first quarter rather than the entire year. According to predictions by Bloomberg Economics, the global economy might face a loss of 0.416 percentage point in the first quarter of 2020. Deeply conjoint to China in terms of finance, logistics and merchandise, Hong Kong is one of the most likely countries to be affected by the virus.

Slowing down of China means less product exports, which would affect the main product exporters such as Brazil and Australia. Mostly dependent on China in its intermediate goods, South Korea's economic growth in the first quarter of the year might end up 0.4 percentage point, less than expected due to the virus.

Owing to the deficiencies in intermediate good supplies coming from China, a South Korean automobile company decided to halt its operations for some time. Problems to be caused by the virus and a breakdown in expectations in the global supply chain are expected to negatively impact the U.S. and various EU countries. Among the EU countries, the virus is expected to affect German economy the most.

Possible impacts on Turkish economy

Since the dependency of Turkish economy on China is less compared to other G20 countries, the impact of Wuhan virus on Turkey might be relatively less. The loss of acceleration in global economic growth and trading volumes might also slow down the growth of export rates in Turkey. On the other hand, Turkey's foreign trade deficit to China might become tighter. A decrease in global growth expectations also brings down the petroleum prices. The petroleum prices dropping below 55 dollars is a positive development in terms of inflation and account balances.

Being limited, this kind of cash inflow would still have positive consequences in the markets. If the expectations about the impact of the virus on the global economy further deteriorate, significant central banks such as FED and ECB could go for an additional monetary expansion.

Such a policy move, although limited, would give Turkey more room to play in terms of interest and currency markets. The final and concrete outcomes of the current possible (positive and negative) impacts will be dependent on which actors are stronger and more influential in the process.

The riskiest scenarios

There are three risky scenarios that might increase the impact of the virus on the global economy. The first significant risk is the possibility to not be able to get the virus under total control by the end of the second quarter of the year. As the weather temperatures increase, the possibility of the virus losing its durability might result in this scenario to not happen.

The growing social tension in China due to the virus and the Beijing government overreacting to this situation is another risky scenario. Although some criticize this, it is obvious that China is acting in a more transparent manner compared to its reaction to SARS outbreak in 2003. In such a serious situation, it is not easy to keep all related issues under control — first and most important of which are quarantine processes.

In this regard, the Beijing government has done relatively a good job until now. If a similar situation were to happen in a Western country, it would not be that easy to keep the situation under control as such. Therefore, the possibility of social tension growing and things getting out of control of the Beijing government is low at present.

The third risky scenario may emerge if Beijing misses the import product total that it guaranteed to buy from the U.S. within the framework of the first phase agreement, which would result in a blunt reaction from U.S. President Donald Trump (such as the threat of raising the tariffs again).

In his statement on the issue last week, Trump emphasized that he would comply by the requirements of the deal and that he has full faith in China overcoming the virus crisis.

We have witnessed Trump suddenly changing his mind on lots of issues countless times. It would not be wise to trust him in this issue entirely. No one can guarantee that he will not outmaneuver China and use this situation in his benefit for the 2020 election campaign.

CORONAVIRUS A BLACK SWAN FOR MARKET, BUT NO MAJOR IMPACT ON INDIAN ECONOMY: EXPERTS

The good news is that the recovery rates are showing signs of improvement worldwide, and the encouraging news that the coronavirus does not survive under conditions of higher temperatures.

Coronavirus outbreak is a black swan event for markets, but is not a major threat to India's economy, experts and brokerages said.

The concerns over the impact of coronavirus on economic growth have kept the markets across the globe jittery.

The good news is that the recovery rates are showing signs of improvement worldwide, and the encouraging news that the coronavirus does not survive under the conditions of higher temperatures.

For India, this is a relief as the winter is drawing to a close.

The epidemic is seen as a black swan event by brokerages and analysts, and they believe that the slowdown in China will have a ripple effect across the globe, and to a certain extent, equity markets are factoring that in.

Experts and brokerages are of the view that supply disruptions due to travel ban, global commodity price movements, levels of inventory, etc. are factors that will impact companies from India Inc.

"The cases of Covid-19 have outnumbered all of the previous pandemics and at a much higher rate of change. Although the fatality rate is the lowest, the ramification of such a virus infecting the production hub and trading partner of the world could have a cascading effect on the global supply chain," said brokerage firm Centrum Broking.

Centrum also highlighted while SARS affected the global economy for a few quarters but the impact was short-lived and the global economy recovered soon, but this time around, the situation remains quite grave as the outbreak occurs at the time when the global economy is already undergoing a slowdown.

A threat or opportunity for India?

China has a prominent role in global economic growth with strong trade linkages with emerging markets. Any disruption in Chinese economic activity is most likely to have significant ramifications on the global economy.

However, this is also an opportunity for India to fill in the gap and find ways to reduce its dependency on imports from China.

"Imports of parts from China would certainly be affected for a while due to coronavirus, but at the same time, there is an opportunity for Indian companies to fill in the gap left behind by their Chinese counterparts," EA Sundaram, Executive Director & CIO- Equities- o3 Capital, said in an interview with Moneycontrol.

On the other hand, Kotak Institutional Equities highlighted that India is relatively immune to a slowdown in Chinese activity as China constitutes 14 percent of its imports and 5 percent of its exports.

"Imports from China are mostly in electrical, electronics, chemicals, plastics and metals sectors while exports to China are concentrated mostly in chemicals, petroleum products, ores and fish. Companies will be able to tide over in the near-term, though prolonged production stoppages will have supply risks for import-dependent sectors," Kotak said. However, the possibility of a prolonged production stoppages looks overdone. Covid-19 has caused large-scale quarantines across China but the outbreak has predominantly been contained in Hubei province, which accounts for 1.3 percent of the total exports of China. Besides, recent reports suggest a declining trend in new cases.

India's consumer durables, electronics, chemicals and pharmaceuticals are high-risk sectors. However, if the cases of coronavirus continue to fall, India need not worry much.

"We believe that the macro impact as a fallout of disruptions in China will be limited assuming the Covid-19 spread stabilizes hereon, and large exporting hubs in China remain relatively less affected," said Kotak.

On February 19, RBI Governor Shaktikanta Das said that the coronavirus outbreak will have a limited impact on India but the global GDP and trade will definitely get affected due to the large size of the Chinese economy.

"Only a couple of sectors in India are likely to see some disruptions but alternatives are being explored to overcome those issues," PTI reported him saying so.

CORONAVIRUS BEGINS TO SPREAD ECONOMIC GLOOM WORLDWIDE

The cascading economic impact of the new coronavirus outbreak in China is becoming more apparent worldwide, with Apple's surprise cut to its sales forecast due to supply chain disruptions spooking global markets and Asian governments downgrading growth prospects. German investor sentiment, meanwhile, is collapsing amid fears the outbreak will kneecap the incipient recovery in global manufacturing.

The fallout from the outbreak of the virus and China's efforts to contain it—with more than 70,000 known cases and more than 1,800 deaths so far—comes at a particularly bad time for economies like Japan and Germany, which were just beginning to recover after a year of global trade tensions weighed on their manufacturing and exports. The virus has hit the global automotive industry particularly hard, which has a nasty knock-on effect not just inside China but also in Japan, South Korea, Germany—and potentially even the United States.

Despite China's insistence that the rate of new infections is stabilizing, alongside an ostensible return to business earlier this month, the economic damage is most apparent inside China. Some sectors, like automobiles, are still all but shuttered as factories deal with worker absences and supply chain shortages and most car dealers remain closed. Other sectors, including mining, travel, construction, and retail, are also taking a big hit as Chinese consumers and workers, limited by travel restrictions and fears of infection, have halted most of their usual activity. "It seems increasingly likely that February will prove to be an economic write-off for China," said the commodities consultancy Wood Mackenzie in a note.

Most forecasters expected the Chinese economy to take a big hit to growth in the first quarter before recovering—thanks to government-fueled stimulus—later in the year. But sentiment about China's growth prospects is souring: The new Bank of America fund managers survey shows top investors expect Chinese GDP growth rates to stabilize just over 5 percent per year for the next three years, a big drop from last year's already sluggish 6 percent and a far cry from the halcyon days of double-digit growth less than a decade ago.

Chinese recovery could prove elusive despite Beijing's efforts to boost lending and lower interest rates, Wood Mackenzie said.

Small and medium-sized businesses were meant to keep paying salaries for absent workers during the shutdown, but many won't be able to as their own revenues are squeezed. That means less disposable income for consumers down the road—turning what should have been a temporary pause in domestic demand for consumer goods into potential permanent demand destruction, the consultancy said.

And even though most of the virus infections and deaths have occurred inside China, the economic fallout is becoming increasingly visible among its Asian neighbors. On Tuesday, South Korean President Moon Jae-in essentially declared an economic emergency, calling for desperate measures to limit the damage to an economy deeply intermeshed with China's. Singapore, for its part, slashed its growth outlook this year and is planning a multibillion-dollar stimulus package to offset lost economic activity. Thailand and Malaysia, too, have cut their own growth expectations, and Malaysia is planning an economic stimulus of its own to contain the damage.

But Japan, which has the most virus cases outside China, might be facing the biggest challenges after an already dismal fourth quarter showed a shrinking economy, with the biggest contraction in more than five years. Japanese automakers like Toyota and Nissan have seen output disrupted both at Chinese factories and at home, while inbound Chinese tourism is paralyzed for now. That raises the real risk of a recession for Japan, which just launched a huge economic stimulus package late last year and may need to prime the pump even further to avoid a full-blown crisis.

Even further afield, the virus is taking its toll. Chinese companies working on projects for the Belt and Road Initiative around Southeast Asia will almost certainly suffer delays and higher costs as supply-chain and worker disruptions percolate through to projects on the ground. Brazil, which relies on the Chinese market as its largest trading partner, will likely see slower growth this year due to the fallout from the outbreak. And, of course, the slowdown will likely derail U.S. plans to massively increase exports of farm produce, energy, and manufactured goods to China, which could delay any real recovery in the distressed Farm Belt and Rust Belt.

And Europe, too, is starting to worry. European automakers such as Volkswagen have already seen production affected at factories inside China, and now there are growing concerns of additional supply chain disruptions that could affect manufacturing in European plants.

Investors in Germany fear the worst, after a dismal year for Europe's biggest economy, mired in a manufacturing slump thanks to a dire outlook for its key auto sector. On Tuesday, the ZEW survey of German investors showed a collapse in sentiment, with fears that the virus and its knock-on effects in China will upend global trade and hamstring Germany's export-led recovery.

The gloomy outlook briefly sent the euro to almost three-year lows against the dollar—which, given U.S. President Donald Trump's constant tirades against unfair competition from lesser-valued foreign currencies, only threatens to ratchet up trans-Atlantic trade tensions even further.

U.S.-CHINA COOPERATION ON CORONAVIRUS AND GLOBAL DISORDER

As Washington and Beijing wage war against the new coronavirus, they are also fighting a public relations battle against each other—one that could expand into a broader conflict that would serve neither country's interests. The opening salvos were fired in early January 2020, as the virus's spread became apparent. Beijing criticized Washington for implementing restrictive travel bans, calling it an "overreaction." Washington rightly censured Beijing for covering up the virus's initial spread and not being transparent with the world, but also used careless language to say the outbreak could be an opportunity for U.S. businesses.

At the time, these developments foreshadowed a further downturn in relations during a devastating viral outbreak. As we wrote in February, "U.S.-China collaboration to eradicate the coronavirus is a chance for both countries to demonstrate they can still cooperate in times of crisis. There are compelling humanitarian and moral reasons for both sides to look past their differences and work together. . . . But the climate in both capitals today indicates that this may not be the case anymore."

China, for now at least, appears to be emerging from the worst of the crisis. President Xi Jinping's visit to the epicenter of the pandemic in Wuhan, rumors that a new date for China's annual Two Session meeting has been set for late April or early May, and even the arrival of Pakistan's president in Beijing last week signal a renewed confidence from Chinese leadership. Now that COVID-19, the disease caused by the new coronavirus, is better controlled within China, Beijing is shifting needed resources abroad. The Foreign Ministry announced it was sending medical equipment to hard-hit countries like South Korea, Iran, and Iraq, and China has sent two teams of medical professionals to assist Italy. Yet China's nascent rebound has exacerbated hostilities with the United States even beyond the trade and economic realm. Most recently, Washington and Beijing began methodically expelling each other's journalists. China escalated that feud on March 18 with an unprecedented ban on reporters from the *New York Times*, the *Wall Street Journal*, and the *Washington Post*.

Meanwhile, Beijing has launched an active public relations campaign to say the virus did not originate in China. Chinese embassies are being instructed to assign the virus labels after other countries, such as the "Italian virus," in an attempt to counter references to the "Wuhan virus." Ministry of Foreign Affairs Spokesperson and newly appointed Deputy Director of China's Foreign Ministry Information Department Zhao Lijian has also repeatedly claimed the virus may have originated in the United States or even been brought to China by the U.S. military. A tweet of Zhao's propagating that claim has been shared by Chinese ambassadors in Cameroon, France, Iran, Jordan, Pakistan, the Philippines and other countries.

These attempts have not gone unnoticed in Washington. Chinese Ambassador to the United States Cui Tiankai was summoned to the State Department to explain Zhao's actions. In a call between U.S. Secretary of State Mike Pompeo and Chinese Director of the Office of Foreign Affairs Yang Jiechi, Pompeo "conveyed strong U.S. objections to [People's Republic of China] efforts to shift blame for COVID-19 to the United States."

The U.S. administration is right to adamantly push back on China's unvalidated claims. As Rush Doshi, director of the Brookings China Strategy Initiative, has argued, "China wants to claim leadership of the global coronavirus response . . . but covering up the virus and brazenly lying about its origins complicates the effort."

For the most part, however, the United States has only succeeded in stoking the flames. Despite pleas from the director of the Centers for Disease Control and Prevention not to adopt geographic labels such as "Chinese coronavirus," senior officials continue to do so. Pompeo consistently refers to the "Wuhan virus," and President Donald Trump tweets about the "Chinese Virus." This is in addition to gratuitously and frequently referencing China as the virus's source in press conferences. According to a recent report, the administration is also rolling out a communications plan to better coordinate talking points and responses for China-related questions, focusing the blame for the outbreak squarely on Beijing.

Washington cannot and should not stand for false statements made by Beijing. But it also cannot allow itself to be goaded by Beijing's propaganda machine, particularly now that the Chinese have been emboldened by Trump's initial mismanagement of the virus's spread in the United States.

CHINA'S COVID-19 PUSH FOR GLOBAL INFLUENCE

The coronavirus pandemic is a "black swan" moment. It is a rare and unpredictable event that could have momentous, system-wide, and unforeseen consequences. China deserves credit for having mobilised quickly, efficiently, and effectively after initial missteps to defeat the COVID-19 disease. Domestically, the early cover-ups and punishment of whistle-blowers have been displaced by the narrative of a heroic patriotic victory led by President Xi Jinping and the Chinese Communist Party.

Beijing is now retooling to capitalise by claiming global leadership on turning the tide. While many Western countries dithered, China successfully contained the epidemic with efficiency as a strong state.

Meanwhile, India is using equally brutal tactics to enforce the world's harshest lockdown, for example, by spraying desperate migrant workers with chemical disinfectant. The privileged jet-setters who imported the virus can utilise the private hospitals but the poor they infect have little access to decent health care and will be disproportionately devastated.

One roadblock to Beijing's global lustre is the aggressive questioning of why greater China has been the source of many serial flu outbreaks. Even the 1918 "Spanish Flu" pandemic may have started with Chinese labourers.

China must implement tough measures to clean up the wet markets that are breeding grounds for species-hopping viruses. "National sovereignty" is a meaningless juridical fiction against the empirical reality of diseases that cross borders at lightning speed.

The four-decade rise of China has greatly enhanced its weight in regional and global institutions, and also cemented its place as the hub of global supply chains across a broad array of manufacturing sectors. The pandemic highlighted the world's dependence on China for critical supplies as a risk with a concreteness that no amount of abstract discussions could capture.

Policies will henceforth pivot, on strategic grounds, to self-reliance and diversification of suppliers. However, this must be supplemented with building international functional redundancy in food supplies, health and value chains in a deliberate strategy of reducing risk through diversification.

The financial crisis of 2008 to 2009 marked the end of the "unipolar" moment of unchallengeable US primacy. China skilfully exploited the collapse of US and European reputation for economic competence and moral and financial rectitude to expand its worldwide soft power. The coronavirus panic could potentially mark the moment of Chinese ascendancy in the "psychological balance of power".

Will voters reward US President Donald Trump for his intuition that US trade policies had facilitated the rise of China as a potentially hostile great power and given it the tools to disrupt the supplies of essential goods in a global emergency?

Trump seems uninterested in exercising US diplomatic and economic leadership. The European Union has failed the test in its responses to Italy, an original member, and Serbia, a candidate country.

Serbia was encouraged to switch imports from China to Europe but was refused medical goods to cope with COVID-19 because the equipment is needed for EU health care systems; Italy issued urgent requests for ventilators and masks, but none were forthcoming from EU partners.

China stepped into the breach in both cases, complete with photo-ops.

China's diplomatic march through developing countries, where the biggest killer is poverty, will be even more decisive. The world's bottom billion subsist in a Hobbesian state of nature where life is "nasty, brutish and short".

The human and economic costs of coronavirus will be far more devastating with low state capacity, weak health systems, teeming slums, unclean water and sanitation systems, congested mass transit, and inadequate safety nets. The killer ailments are water-borne infectious diseases, nutritional deficiencies and neonatal and maternal complications.

The biggest death toll from the 1918 pandemic – between one-sixth and one-third of the total – was in India.

Coronavirus threatens to overwhelm the health and economies of many developing countries dependent on tourism and commodity exports and vulnerable to capital flight. In addition to lending a helping hand to Italy and Serbia, China, Jack Ma and the Alibaba Foundation have also shipped supplies to countries in Asia, the Middle East and Africa.

Exploiting the open lack of Euro-Atlantic solidarity, China has waged a surprisingly successful coronavirus narrative war as the world's white knight. The US and European governments have focused inwardly on domestic concerns; China has kept its eye on the prize of discrediting and displacing the US as the go-to major power in global crises.

Most recipient countries of China's largesse to help cope with the pandemic will soften criticisms of its domestic and regional misdemeanours.

With US disengagement from the UN, China has put its nationals at the head of four of the UN's 15 specialised agencies, compared to other Security Council permanent members with just one each.

In a compelling demonstration of the consequences of the crumbling architecture of world order, Trump's disruption of the global trading order made it correspondingly more difficult to organise a coordinated response to the pandemic or to provide the requisite world leadership.

Amidst the potential wreckage of the major Western economies under protracted lockdowns, China's capital markets remain strong and far from fearing a decoupled world, China may set the terms on which it's implemented.

In fresh proof that history does irony, the coronavirus epidemic that was "Made in China" and multiplied out of control because of initial obfuscation and denialism, may end up expanding China's global reach and influence.

8

Coronavirus : Impact on Chinese and Indian Economy

Coronavirus: Economists are comparing 2019-nCoV to SARS epidemic of 2002-03. While India could have been insulated from the economic impact back then, it is near impossible to do that in today's age

Novel coronavirus: With the declaration of coronavirus (2019-nCoV) as a global emergency, the entire world is likely to feel the impact of the massive outbreak that has claimed many lives and infected over 48,000 people in China alone.

The impact could have a ripple effect on all major economies across the world, particularly in the manufacturing sector, since most of them depend on Chinese imports to complete their assembly line.

India's Minister of Health, Dr. Harsh Vardhan, in a press briefing said, "We had declared the novel coronavirus as a health emergency on January 17 itself. In all our airports thermal screening has been activated. The figures from China are: 48,206 affected cases, 1310 deaths. There are 28 countries that are impacted, if we consider Hong Kong, Taiwan and Macau as separate."

Some economists in India believe that this is not the time to gloat over China's problems or look at opportunities but to offer help and assistance in real terms since the impact will be felt in India very soon. Speaking to India Today, Mohan Guruswamy said, "One economy's shutdown doesn't benefit another. When global markets slow down, all of us get hit. China today accounts for one-sixth of the global GDP. Seventy per cent of manufacturing exports are from China. Wait for a few months, there will be a global slump. Pharmaceuticals, rare minerals, etc come from China. Slowdown will start affecting everybody."

The major sectors that would be impacted are automobile sector, pharmaceuticals and technology hardware sector since most of the parts for these products are made in China and all essential chemicals in the pharma sector come from China to India.

According to reports, Hyundai decided to shut down three of its South Korean plants due to shortages of a wiring harness that was no longer available from a supplier in China. If this continues then Indian markets will also be hit severely.

The real brunt of it has not been felt yet since the outbreak happened during the Chinese lunar holiday. With around 7 million workers, mostly assembly line workers slated to return, one will have to see if they would be allowed to resume work.

Wuhan is a major production centre. Hubei province as a whole is a manufacturing hub. With these factories shutting shop, assembly lines will shut down in places like Shanghai, if even one part does not reach them.

Economists are comparing 2019-nCoV to SARS epidemic of 2002-03. While India could have been insulated from the economic impact back then, it is near impossible to do that in today's age.

"The rest of Asia will not be immune to the spillover effects from China, as it's economically more deeply integrated with China today than during SARs 17 years ago," Nomura, an Asia-headquartered financial services group, said in a recent note.

The only advantage that India has, according to Mohan Guruswamy, is that manufacturers store raw material because of India's "inefficient" systems. So, while India may not witness the hit immediately, she will in due course.

CORONAVIRUS: INDIA INC WILL SHIVER IF CHINA CAN'T CONTAIN OUTBREAK

India's economic woes could amplify as many of the country's key sectors rely heavily on components or parts manufactured in China.

Growing insecurity over the coronavirus (Covid-19) epidemic in China may have a sharp impact on India's already-strained economy as industries fear that the outbreak could cripple their production activities.

A recent report by Ind-RA said efforts to contain the virus outbreak within next three to four months will be critical as it would determine the fate of many industries around the globe, including in India. If the virus is contained within the aforesaid time period, the impact on businesses in India and elsewhere will not be overgenerous, the report said.

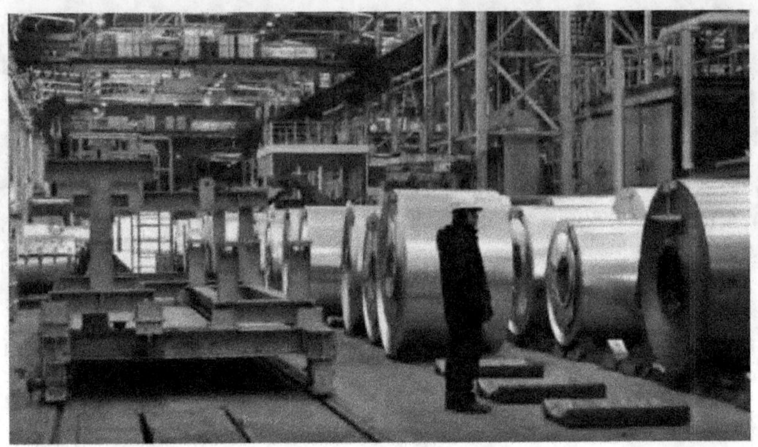

But if no positive result comes within a few months, multiple Indian sectors could face major supply-side disturbances, triggering a delay in key manufacturing activities. The Ind-Ra report goes on to highlight that the economic impact could be worse than what was seen during the SARS outbreak in 2003. At that time, the world was less dependent on China, now considered the biggest world's biggest manufacturing hub with a substantial contribution to the global GDP.

China now contributes to over one-sixth or over 15 per cent of the world's GDP and any deceleration in manufacturing activity could significantly impact worldwide growth.

Commenting on the situation, Sunil Damania, CIO, MarketsMojo.com, said, "For some reason, if China is unable to control it for six months, the impacts would be severe."

"It's very difficult to quantify as there are many moving parts. But it would have a significant impact and has the potential to drag down the world's GDP growth rate by at least 20 basis points for CY2020," he added.

Impact On India

The Indian economy is already battling many headwinds including inflation, slow demand, and lower-income, which resulted in a sharp fall in GDP growth in 2019. Economic woes could amplify as many of the country's key sectors rely heavily on components or parts manufactured in China.

While the government predicted India's growth for the next fiscal at 6.5 per cent, delay in supply of key essential commodities from China for a prolonged period could spill water on that optimistic forecast.

Some sectors such as automobiles, consumer electronics, drugs and pharmaceuticals — all of which contribute significantly to the country's GDP — will bear the brunt of the supply curbs. Interlinked sectors will also suffer as a result. "If the outbreak continues for longer than anticipated then the risk will not be restricted to a few sectors, but it can hurt the overall economy," Damania said. Some industry experts said trade has already been mildly affected in India as supply chain issues start cropping up. The impact will start showing when firms run out of inventory, they said.

Lower Jobs, Inflation And More

A delay in the supply of inventory would not only lead to lower production but will also lower sales volume. It could also lead to job cuts and higher inflation.

For instance, many electronic goods and phone manufacturers have already started facing the effects of supply slowdown as companies in China failed to restart key manufacturing activities. Major smartphone sellers like Xiaomi hinted at possible rise in prices as supplies of key components are already facing delays.

A host of Indian smartphone manufacturers, who dearly depend on China for key components, are already indicating that their productions will fall if the supply disruptions continue. It could be a huge blow to India, which is the second-largest smartphone market in the world.

Some analysts are expecting a drop in production and sales of consumer durables and smartphones while others fear that prices could go up in a situation where there is high demand but lack of supply.

Consumer durables like television, washing machines and air conditioners — all of which need critical components manufactured in China — may also see a drop in sales due to lack of supply. What's worse is the fact that it could lead to higher inflationary pressure on India as China vendors have hiked prices of critical components amid the shortage. Higher inflation in times of slow growth could be disastrous for India and could severely disrupt plans to revive the economy.

Like smartphones, automobile manufacturers also import a host of parts and essential components from China. It may be noted that more than 60 per cent of Chinese auto assembly production units have been directly affected by the coronavirus epidemic.

A Boston Consulting Group report said the impact on the Chinese automobile industry will affect many other countries including India. A Fitch report said India's auto production activity could dip by over 8 per cent in 2020 due to the situation.

"China supplies India with between 10-30 per cent of its automotive components and this could be two to three times higher when looking at India's EV segment, which highlights just how exposed India's automobile manufacturing industry is to the slowdown of vehicle Chinese component manufacturing," it said. But manufacturers in India have little choice apart from monitoring the situation and hoping for factories in China to fire up their assembly lines. Some Chinese factories reopened this week, but workers are in no position to resume activities with no solution in sight.

Another concern that India could face due to the virus outbreak in China is job cuts. With lower scope of production activities, some companies will be forced to lay off contractual labourers. This could have a negative effect on India's declining income levels.

Lower manufacturing and production activity due to the virus outbreak could pull down India's Industrial output, which is also not in good shape. To sum it up, a fall in manufacturing output along with ticking inflation and supply constraints could worsen India's growth outlook further.

At the time of writing this chapter, the death toll from the coronavirus outbreak stood at 1,488 with a sharp jump in the number of confirmed cases at over 65,000.

The situation in China remains critical with 121 news deaths on Friday while Japan registered its first death, the third fatality outside China.

Coronavirus impact China's trade: India to benefit in apparel

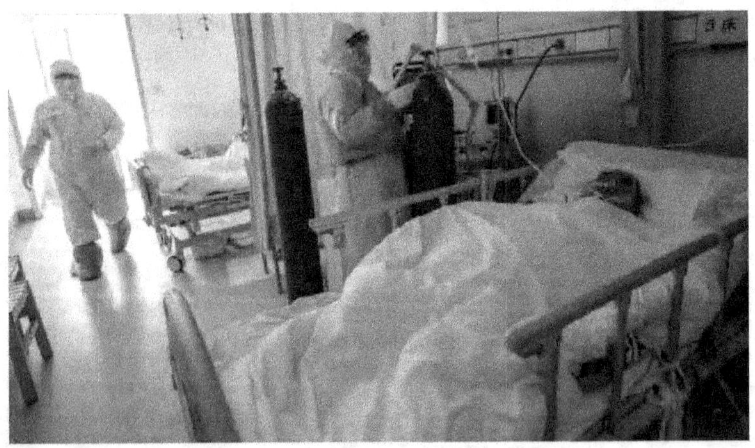

Medical workers provide treatment to a new coronavirus patient at a hospital in Wuhan in central China's Hubei province.

India is expected to be a preferred market for sourcing of apparel products for buyers from the US, UK Europe and Canada as trade with China had been affected due to the novel coronavirus epidemic, Apparel Export Promotion Council Chairman A.Shakivel said on Wednesday.

Countries which had been depending on China have learnt a lesson they should have an alternative market for sourcing and India was expected to be their preferred destination since the Dragon nation's trade had been hit hard, he said. Besides, UK's exit from the European Union would also give an edge to India, he said in a release summing up the three-day 47th edition of India Knit Fair, which concluded at nearby hosiery town of Tirupur.

Shaktivel, who is also the Chairman of the fair, said it was organised in the backdrop of current economic scenario.

Tamil Nadu Handlooms and Textiles Director M Karunakaran, who was present on the inaugural day, said the state's Textile Policy would support the growth of knitting and textile sector. The fair featured summer and winter collections in knitwear for all age groups, including infants, along with cotton, polyester, polycotton, Polyester-viscose blended fabric apparels, Shaktivel said.

Specially made garments made from banana cotton, blend with 80 per cent cotton and 20 per cent banana fibre, attracted visitors.

As many as 31 buyers and 142 buying house and agents from different countries visited the stalls during the fair which was expected to generate business worth Rs 300 crore, he said. A total of 39 leading exporters from Tiruppur, Coimbatore, Chennai, and Kolkatta participated and displayed their products.

CORONAVIRUS IN INDIA: HOW THE 2019-NCOV COULD IMPACT THE FAST-GROWING ECONOMY

Since the Wuhan coronavirus outbreak in China, the highest number of suspected cases in India has been reported in the state of Kerala. Suspected coronavirus cases have also been reported in multiple cities such as New Delhi, Mumbai, Bengaluru, Hyderabad, and Patna. The current coronavirus situation in India remains stable, with no new cases reported.

Coronavirus cases in India: Confirmed, suspected and recovered

A total of 1,671 suspected cases have been tested and three confirmed cases have been reported in India. All the three with confirmed coronavirus are from Kerala and have been discharged, but home-quarantined.

Indians on quarantined cruise ship Diamond Princess

The latest coronavirus cases in India are reported from the Diamond Princess cruise ship quarantined off the coast of Yokohama in Japan. A total of 12 people from India have tested positive for the virus on the ship as of 24 February. The infected persons are reported to be a stable condition. A total of 132 passengers and six crew members from India are reportedly on board the ship.

The Indian Embassy is working towards disembarking all Indian nationals on board the ship.

Coronavirus disease in India: Approved treatments

The Drug Controller General of India has granted approval to the Indian Council of Medical Research to use a combination of lopinavir and ritonavir in the event of the coronavirus disease in India turns into a public health emergency, reported the Economic Times. Lopinavir and ritonavir have already been approved for the treatment of HIV.

Covid-19: Measures India has taken to control the Wuhan coronavirus spread

Evacuation measures

The Indian government arranged for the evacuation of 366 Indian citizens from Wuhan in a special Air India flight on 31 January 2020. The passengers are placed under quarantine for a period of 14 days.

A second batch of passengers, including seven Maldivan citizens evacuated by the government, arrived from Wuhan on 01 February 2020. The repatriated passengers are currently being monitored. India evacuated 645 people by 11 February. The health condition of all of them is being monitored on a daily basis.

The Indian embassy announced plans for a special flight to Wuhan on 17 February that will carry medical supplies and return with Indians citizens who wish to return to the country.

Visas cancelled for foreign nationals travelling from China

India announced cancellation of existing visas issued to all foreign nationals travelling from China, on 05 February and advised Indians to avoid travelling to China.

Further, India announced that people travelling to China will be quarantined upon return.

Coronavirus screening, testing and quarantining at Indian airports

Thermal screening has been installed at 21 airports including those in Delhi, Mumbai, Kolkata, Chennai, Bengaluru, Hyderabad, and Cochin to check for coronavirus in India. Universal screening has been mandated for flights from China, Hong Kong, Singapore and Thailand at the aero-bridges ear-marked for the purpose.

Travellers with symptoms of the infection are being separated by the Ministry of Health & Family Welfare's Integrated Disease Surveillance Programme (IDSP) and directed to isolation facilities. The IDSP has been testing their samples.

The Ministry of Health announced on 06 February that all 645 evacuees from Wuhan tested negative. Two quarantine centres have been set-up to isolate any passengers showing symptoms of the infection. One centre is located at Manesar, Haryana, and is managed by Armed Forces Medical Services, while the second is located at Chawla Camp in Delhi and is managed by Indo-Tibetan Border Police (ITBP).

A total of 406 evacuees who were quarantined at the ITBP facility were discharged and allowed to return home on 19 February.

Labs testing for coronavirus in India

The National Institute of Virology, Pune, and ten other laboratories under the Indian Council of Medical Research's (ICMR) Viral Research and Diagnostics Laboratories network are equipped to test samples.

The ICMR has tested 510 samples as of 06 February, of which three tested positive, according to the latest coronavirus update in India.

Travel restrictions by India in the wake of Covid-19

The Indian government issued a travel advisory on 17 January 2020 to the general public to refrain from travelling to China and avoid contact with anyone with travel history to China since 15 January 2020.

The government also temporarily suspended e-Visa facility for Chinese passport holders and noted that already issued e-Visas are temporarily invalid. Online application for physical visa from China has also been suspended.

Any persons trying to visit India under compelling circumstances have been advised to contact either the Indian embassy in Beijing or the Indian consulate in Shanghai or Guangzhou.

Coronavirus impact on India

Impact on India's trade with China

With China under lockdown, India is expected to witness a major impact on imports and exports in various industries including pharmaceuticals, electronics, mobiles, and auto parts.

China is the biggest exporter to India, followed by the US and UAE. In 2018, China exported goods worth $90.4bn to India and accounted for 14.63% of the exports.

In 2017, telecom instruments, electronics components, computer hardware and peripherals, industrial machinery for dairy, and organic chemicals were the top five items imported by India accounting for 46% of the imports from China.

How the Covid-19 outbreak impacts the Indian pharmaceutical industry

Bulk drugs and drug intermediates accounted for $1.5bn or 3% of India's imports from China. According to the Trade Promotion Council of India, approximately 85% of active pharmaceutical ingredients (APIs) imported by Indian companies are from China. India's overdependence on China for APIs exposes it to raw material supply disruption and price volatility. Another major hindrance to the Indian pharmaceutical industry is its low capacity utilisation, according to a report from the Ministry of Commerce and Industry (MCI). India has a capacity utilisation between 30% and 40% as against 75% of China.

Opportunities for Indian pharmaceutical manufacturers

Although the Wuhan coronavirus outbreak could have a significant impact on the Indian pharmaceutical industry unless it is brought under control over the next few months, it also provides an opportunity to India's pharmaceutical manufacturers to grab share from their Chinese competitors.

Indian pharmaceutical companies currently have two months' stock of APIs and intermediates, quoted the Economic Times. In the absence of a major disruption due to the outbreak, the existing stocks may address the issue of shortage, it added.

The report from MCI, however, noted that improving the overall capacity utilisation of existing manufacturing plants in India as a short-term solution to such supply disruptions. The report noted the need for assured purchase agreements from the government for the existing manufacturing plants.

It also noted that the government should absorb the price differential to improve capacity utilisation.

Export ban on protection equipment

The Directorate General of Foreign Trade issued a ban on the export of personal protection equipment such as respiratory masks and protective overalls, on 31 January. The exact reason for the ban has not been notified, though.

HOW WILL CHINA'S CORONAVIRUS SHUTDOWN AFFECT INDIAN ECONOMY

Shutdown at Hubei, a major component hub, might have far-reaching consequences. As China is busy fighting the deadly coronavirus, it is speculated that the Lunar New Year holiday might be extended, at least in certain provinces, till February 17 from February 10. The news of a possible extend of shutdown is sending shivers across the world as these provinces have a greater share in China's and, in effect, the global economy, including India.

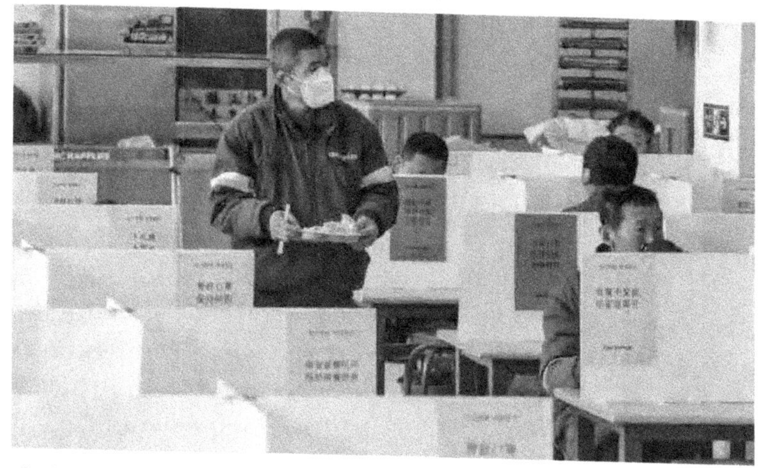

Millions of people in China were returning to work on February 10 after an extended holiday designed to slow the spread of the new coronavirus, which has killed more than 900 people

For instance, the 11 Chinese provinces which have announced an extended holiday period are normally responsible for over two-third of vehicle production in China, with projected crisis-induced first quarter production loss of around 350,000 units if they are idled until February 10, 2020. If the situation lingers into mid-March, and plants in adjacent provinces are also idled, the China-wide supply chain disruption caused by parts shortages from Hubei, a major component hub, could have a wide-reaching impact.

Automobile

India largely sources electronics, engineering goods, and chemicals from China. Non-availability of such products from China would mean related parties in India will have to scout for alternative markets, which can mean higher costs.

This will undoubtedly have far-reaching consequences for India's automobile sector as well. Already battling one of the worst slowdowns in over two decades, the virus attack would mean further doom for India's auto sector. According to Maruti Chairman R.C. Bhargava, many Maruti vendors in India rely on supplies of components and raw materials from China. "Most of them have inventories of up to 30 days. Total imports are small, but the point is that for a car, even if one component is not there, I can't put the car on the road," he told *CNBC* recently. The shortage will force manufacturers and vendors to scout for alternative sources of supply, which will probably add to the cost of making a car.

Travel and tourism

Another sector that might reel under the coronavirus attack is travel and tourism. In 2019, Chinese accounted for 3.12 per cent of the total foreign tourist arrivals in India. Arrival of toursists from China have increased over the years in India. However, that might see a reversal this year, at least in the first. The travel advisory against China will also dampen the aviation industry. IndiGo, which operated three routes from India to China, have temporarily suspended service on two routes. Air India, too, has halted operations to China.

Trade

China is India's biggest trading partner. The country accounted for 14 per cent of Indian imports in 2018-19. The Communist party-led country also accounted for 5 per cent of India's exports in the same year, making it the third-largest market for domestic goods. "The disruption caused, if prolonged, could have a bearing on India's imports from the country which is critical for domestic economic activity. Finding substitutes for imports from China in the near term could be a challenge," noted credit agency CARE Ratings in a recent report. "Further, a slowdown in economic activity in China could impact exports from India."

"On the flip side, the real economic impact of what is happening in China is for real. We are seeing it across sectors. The diamond market is expecting a huge loss. M&M made a statement that some of their models could get impacted. The raw material cost for common drugs like paracetamol cost have doubled in 10 days. Solar power developers are looking to declare force majeure because those things might not come in. The real economic impact will be seen over the next two, three, four months," stock market expert Sandip Sabharwal told *ET*.

In addition, the supply chain of leather industry, which depends on China for components such as soles, and ornaments is likely to get hit.

Opportunity

Even as the threat looms large, China's economic shutdown opens various doors for India. As per a recent report in the *Economic Times*, global buyers are seeing India as China's replacement to source ceramics, homeware, fashion and lifestyle goods, textiles, engineering goods and furniture. Reportedly, Indian manufacturers and exporters have seen rising number of interests from the western market.

Mainland China is now the second-largest importer in the world, accounting for 10.4 per cent of the world's goods imports, compared with 4 per cent of the world's imports in 2002. "With local production being affected (due to the coronavirus outbreak), there could be an increase in China's imports from other countries which can provide an opportunity for Indian manufacturers," the CARE report observed. India mainly exports chemicals, petroleum, agriculture, engineering goods, cotton yarn and plastics to China.

9

Coronavirus in China: The Outbreak, Measures, and Impact on Global Economy

Majority of the deaths caused by the epidemic have been in China among all the countries affected by coronavirus. The first death outside Mainland China occurred in the Philippines soon followed by Hong Kong, Japan, France and Taiwan.

Chinese President Xi Jinping noted that the impact of the outbreak on the country's economy is manageable and advised on the orderly resumption of work on 24 February. He noted that each region in the country should adopt a precise approach keeping in mind the health and safety risks involved.

The highest number of cases in China is in the Hubei province, where the virus is believed to have originated. Within Hubei, the city of Wuhan accounts for the highest number of confirmed cases, followed by Zhejiang, Guangdong, and Hunan. The province registered a 30% spike in new confirmed cases of 14,840 on 13 February 2020. Hubei also reported the highest percentage of deaths as well as the highest percentage of cured patients, among all the coronavirus affected areas in the country.

To contain the spread of the disease, China has temporarily suspended air, road, and rail travel in and out of Wuhan and neighbouring provinces. These restrictions were also placed for airlines based in Hong Kong, Macau, and Taiwan.

Number of new infections decline

China reported a decline in the number of new cases reported for the first time since the outbreak on 18 February. The number of recovered patients at 1,824 surpassed the number of new confirmed cases at 1,749. Anthony S. Fauci, immunologist and director of the National Institute of Allergy and Infectious Diseases, noted that it is too early to determine whether the cases are declined. He added that the trend needs to be followed closely for a few days before concluding that there is a decline.

Restrictions in Xiaogan city – the second-worst affected city in China

People in the Xiaogan city of Hubei province of China have been banned from leaving their homes in an effort to contain the spread of the disease. The Xiaogan city is the second city to report the highest number of cases after Wuhan. As of 18 February, 3,320 confirmed cases and 75 deaths have been reported in the city.

The Xiaogan city is home to more than four million people who will have to remain in their homes or face ten days in detention, if the restrictions are not followed. All vehicles have been banned from roads and public events have been cancelled. Medical workers and people transporting essential goods have been exempt from the restrictions. Few supermarkets and pharmacies are expected to remain open during the ban.

Travel restrictions imposed on Chinese tourists and visitors

Several countries have closed their borders with China, while some have cut direct transportation links, including the US, Australia, New Zealand, Indonesia, Maldives, and Japan.

The World Health Organisation (WHO), however, has advised against imposing any travel or trade restrictions on China, despite declaring the outbreak as a global public health emergency.

Countries that have restricted or banned Chinese tourists or visitors

The US issued the highest level of travel advisory (level 4) on 2 February 2020 and advised its citizens not to travel to China. It also urged US citizens in China to depart by commercial means or stay home as much as possible while avoiding contact with others.

Australia announced enhanced border control measures on 1 February 2020 to contain the spread of the virus. All arriving passengers are subjected to enhanced screening measures and passengers departing China from 1 February 2020 are denied entry into the country. The travel excludes Australian citizens, permanent residents, and their immediate family members.

New Zealand issued temporary travel restrictions into the country for all foreign nationals arriving from China. The restrictions have been placed for up to 14 days and are planned to be reviewed every 48 hours.

Maldives announced new border security measures on 3 February 2020 to restrict entry of all passengers excluding Maldivian citizens from China or those who have transited through China. The country also warned Maldivians against non-essential travel to China and other countries affected by the virus.

Indonesia, Israel, Iraq, Italy, Guatemala, El Salvador Oman, Saudi Arabia, Russia, Japan, Vietnam, Singapore, and Pakistan are some of the other countries that have either imposed travel restrictions or cancelled direct flights to China, as reported by the BBC and Reuters.

How China is responding to the novel coronavirus outbreak

China has taken immediate measures to contain the spread of the virus and provide diagnosis and treatment in-time to reduce the impact.

On 23 January, the Chinese Civil Aviation Administration guided foreign airlines to reduce their scheduled flights to Wuhan, when necessary, to prevent and control the spread of pneumonia caused by coronavirus.

The government has taken a number of measures to contain the outbreak, as listed below:

- Pooling trained medical personnel from across the country
- Ensuring supplies to the most vulnerable and affected areas
- Construction of new hospitals on a war-footing
- Extending holidays for schools and businesses as well as the Chinese Lunar New Year holiday

Cancellation/postponement of events

The Shanghai Fashion Week scheduled to be held between 26 March to 2 April has been cancelled by the organisers due to the COVID-19 outbreak.

Juss Sports Group, promoter of the 2020 Chinese Grand Prix, requested the postponement of the event scheduled to be held between 17 April and 19 April due to health concerns related to COVID-19. Formula One (F1) and Fédération Internationale de l'Automobile (FIA) have accepted the request.

The Chinese Grand Prix is a key part of F1's calendar. Based on how the outbreak situation emerges over the next few months, the Grand Prix event may be rescheduled towards the later part of the year, the FIA noted.

Preventive measures at Chinese airports

Anticipating huge passenger movements on the occasion of the Spring Festival, China closed the outbound traffic from Wuhan, on 25 January, at a time when the coronavirus spread was anticipated to intensify. Screening was started at most airports with flights arriving from Wuhan and other affected areas to admit passengers with associated symptoms for observation, diagnosis, and care.

Building hospitals for coronavirus care and treatment

China preponed the opening of the Dabie Mountain Regional Medical Centre, a 1,000-bed hospital, by expediting its construction and opened it on 29 January to quarantine people with coronavirus symptoms. It also opened a second quarantine hospital named Leishenshan hospital in Wuhan with 1,500 beds.

A new 1,000-bed hospital, named Huoshenshan hospital, was completed in record ten days to provide enhanced care and treatment to coronavirus patients. The new makeshift hospital was opened for admitting patients on 03 February.

China, further, decided to convert 11 venues, across Wuhan city, including gymnasiums, exhibition centres and sports centres into make-shift hospitals with more than 10,000 beds to treat patients with mild symptoms. Eight additional venues were announced to be converted into hospitals. The first three venues were converted on 03 February providing 3,400 beds to treat patients. In addition, 20 mobile hospitals and 1,400 nurses have been deployed from across the country to Wuhan to treat patients with mild symptoms. An infectious disease hospital is also being built in Zhengzhou, Henan Province.

Faster diagnosis and vaccine/drug development efforts

Wuhan Institute of Virology of the Chinese Academy of Sciences developed two diagnostic kits for the novel coronavirus antibody in association with a biopharmaceutical company.

Using an optimised testing method developed by Zhongnan Hospital of Wuhan University, the infection is being diagnosed in just two hours or more, which has helped to start treatment quicker and improve recoveries.

The National Medical Products Administration also approved two diagnostic kits and a testing system developed by Hubei-based biopharmaceutical companies on 26 January.

Meanwhile, vaccine development efforts are progressing, with two chemical compounds having been found to be effective in restraining the viral activity that will help expedite the drug development for the novel coronavirus.

Wuhan Jinyintan Hospital was the first to use Kaletra (lopinavir/ritonavir), a HIV/AIDS drug, to treat the novel coronavirus patients and note that it's working.

The Chinese Academy of Sciences offered Chinese researchers open and free access to the China Science and Technology Cloud (CSTC) resources and services to assist in their research of the 2019-nCoV. Researchers will gain access to high-performance computing and software and other resources to facilitate interaction with co-researchers.

Baidu Research has allowed gene testing agencies, epidemic control centres and research institutions to use LinearFold, its RNA structure algorithm that will help to understand the virus and screening compounds in less than half-a-minute compared to approximately an hour earlier.

Ban on sale of fever and cough medications

China has banned the sale of fever and cough medicine in certain provinces to encourage people to seek medical attention in hospitals rather than self-medicating. Pharmacies across Nanjing and Hangzhou have announced the ban on the sale of medicines, reported CNN.

Pharmacies in Beijing have been instructed to register all customers who purchase fever and cough medicine including their names, addresses, ID card numbers and contact information apart from their symptoms, as reported by state-run news agency Xinhua.

Coronavirus impact on China

The coronavirus outbreak has resulted in closures of multiple air, rail and road routes, as well as production cuts and temporary closures of manufacturing plants, which are expected to shave-off billions of dollars from China's GDP.

Big companies such as Apple closed stores and manufacturing temporarily, while big telecom companies such as Huawei suspended travel to and from China.

Impact on industries

Some of the industries that are expected to be hit by the coronavirus in China are travel and tourism, shipping, pharmaceutical, automobile, electronics, and manufacturing. Supply chain disruptions are expected to affect a number of associated industries and markets.

Data from the China Association of Automobile Manufacturers (CAAM) has revealed that auto sales declined by 18% in January, as reported by Reuters. The outbreak is expected to affect both sales and production in the short term due to the extension of holidays and shortage of workers and auto parts. The CAAM also predicted that competition will intensify in the industry and that suppliers of smaller parts may collapse.

The Hubei province is a major car manufacturing hub for several companies including Dongfeng Motor Group, Honda Motor, Renault SA and Peugeot SA. All the companies have announced that they will be delaying the restart of production. Companies that operate plants outside Hubei including Tesla, Volkswagen, and General Motors also announced that their factories will be closed for the next few weeks. Major companies that have announced a business impact in the coronavirus affected country are Nike, Hyundai, Starbucks, Tata Motors, McDonald's, Disney, Carlsberg, and H&M, as reported by Reuters and CNBC. Airbus closed its final assembly line in Tianjin on 05 February.

Kering, owned by Gucci, announced the temporary closure of half of its stores in China on 12 February owing to the COVID-19 outbreak, reported Reuters.

Impact on the pharmaceutical industry and supply chain

The Chinese pharmaceutical industry is expected to be adversely impacted by the coronavirus on the supply chain side. China accounts for 13% of the active pharmaceutical ingredients manufactured for the US market, according to the FDA, while India accounts for a higher 18%.

Production and logistics delays could cost the Chinese API manufacturers high if the Indian competitors scale-up quickly.

CORONAVIRUS IMPACT ON THE CHINESE ECONOMY

China has enjoyed an average GDP growth rate of 10% in the last 40 years, but the growth rate has been southwards in the recent years due to multiple reasons, especially structural constraints.

Coronavirus has hit at a time when the Chinese economy is slowing down and the nation is struggling to identify new growth drivers amid trade tensions with the US. The World Bank estimated China to record a lower 6.1% growth rate in 2019 and forecast the economic growth to dip below 6% in 2020 and moderate further in 2021.

The coronavirus is expected to result in a further slow down because of its impact on the country's trade and effect on a wide range of industries, although the estimates are yet to be made.

Measures China is taking to minimise the economic impact of coronavirus

China has already taken a number of fiscal measures to reduce the impact of the coronavirus, although the impact on Q1 is imminent and further impact is subject to bringing the epidemic under control.

Fiscal measures: Liquidity infusion and tariff cuts

The People's Bank of China (PBOC) announced plans to perform reverse repurchase operations worth RMB1.2tn ($173bn) to ensure adequate liquidity supply in the economy. The existing liquidity in the banking system is RMB900bn ($129bn), more than that recorded during the same period in the previous year.

The central bank infused 1.7 trillion yuan already into the banking system via repos and repo rate cuts as of 10 February.

China is also likely to announce tariff cuts on essential goods imported from major countries such as the US, to ensure supplies, despite the recent trade war between the two nations.

Further, Chinese provinces and municipalites are taking multiple supportive measures to support businesses, as below:

- Tax and rent deductions to businesses
- Delaying loan payments
- Reducing interest rates
- Waiving overdue interest on loans
- Offering fresh loans to companies having low liquidity

Non-fiscal measures

The government is currently focusing majorly on minimising the epidemic spread and safeguarding the lives of its residents to minimise the death toll.

The Chinese Ministry of Commerce is ensuring to maintain enough supplies of meat, pork and other essential food products, to avoid shortage.

In the upcoming times, the nation is expected to initiate more non-fiscal measures to reduce the economic impact.

CORONAVIRUS BRINGS MORE BAD NEWS FOR INDIA'S BELEAGUERED ECONOMY

The coronavirus outbreak, which has its epicentre in China's Wuhan city, can impact some sectors of India's embattled economy.

China is the country's biggest trading partner, accounting for the largest share (14%) of Indian imports in financial year 2019. It is also the third-largest market for domestic goods, accounting for 5% of India's exports last financial year.

"The disruption caused, if prolonged, could have a bearing on India's imports from the country which is critical for domestic economic activity. Finding substitutes for imports from China in the near term could be a challenge," noted credit agency CARE Ratings in a recent report. "Further, a slowdown in economic activity in China could impact exports from India."

There have been three confirmed cases of coronavirus in the country so far, all in the southern state of Kerala. The state government, on Feb. 4, declared the fatal disease as a "state calamity."

In China, the disease has claimed 563 lives, so far. Due to the panic, on Feb. 3, Chinese stock markets faced their worst sell-off in many years, wiping out nearly half a trillion dollars from the value of the country's leading firms.

Impact on industries

The hit on the Chinese economy is bound to have a domino effect on a host of sectors in India.

- Tourism: In 2019, India's total foreign tourist arrivals (FTA) stood at 10.9 million, of which Chinese travellers accounted for 3.12%. "Despite it being marginal, FTA share from China has been increasing for the past few years. Therefore the Indian tourism industry is expected to be negatively impacted during 2020," CARE Ratings said in its report.
- Aviation: The sector which could be most impacted is Indian aviation. The outbreak has forced Indian carriers to the cancel and temporarily suspended flights operating from India to China and Hong Kong. Carriers such as Indigo and Air India have halted operations to China.
- Another domestic carrier SpiceJet is offering a waiver of cancellation/change fee for flights booked to China. "The temporary suspension of flights to China and Hong Kong can approximately lead to an Indian carrier missing out on gross revenue of Rs55-72 lakh per flight," CARE stated.
- Bollywood: Due to the outbreak, China has closed nearly 70,000 theatres, according to reports. Recent years have witnessed many Bollywood movies, like *Dangal* and *3 Idiots*, become massive hits in the country and the demand is only growing. Now, many scheduled releases will be impacted due to the fatal virus disease.
- Electronics: About 6-8% of India's exports of electronic goods is to China. Also, around 50-60% of India's demand for electronics is met by China, as per the CARE report. "In FY19, the share of imports of electronic goods from China declined to about 37% from the share of 57% a year ago," it noted. Based on the decreasing dependence in FY19, the report observed that the impact on the electronics good market will be "limited".
- Auto and auto components: India's automobile industry is already struggling with falling sales. Car sales fell 19% last year while sales of two-wheelers declined 14%, Reuters reported. Vehicle makers, including market leader Maruti Suzuki, import components and raw materials from China. However,

Maruti's chairman thinks this will not impact the sector. "It's not a large amount," RC Bhargava told CNBC, referring to the number of components Maruti and its vendors import from China. "Total imports are small, but the point is that for a car, even if one component is not there, I can't put the car on the road."

- The Care Ratings report also echoed Bhargava's opinions. "India's exports of transport equipment to China account for a negligible share of about 0.5% of the total transport equipment exported from the country," it said.
- Besides, the coronavirus outbreak has hit the ongoing Auto Expo 2020 in Delhi. The Indian government had issued an advisory temporarily suspending e-visa facility for Chinese travellers and foreigners, following which, Chinese manufacturers decided to let their Indian representatives man the stalls at the auto expo.

Export opportunity, import crisis

The crisis, though presents an opportunity for Indian exporters.

"With local production being affected (due to the coronavirus outbreak), there could be an increase in China's imports from other countries which can provide an opportunity for Indian manufacturers," the CARE report observed.

India mainly exports chemicals, petroleum, agriculture, engineering goods, cotton yarn and plastics to China.

However, substituting imports from China can be tricky. India largely sources electronics, engineering goods, and chemicals from China. "Non-availability of such products from China would mean related parties in India will have to scout for alternative markets which can mean higher costs," the report added.

CHINA'S ECONOMIC FIGHT AGAINST THE CORONAVIRUS

The coronavirus outbreak that began in the Chinese city of Wuhan has spread across the country and beyond its borders, leaving governments at all levels in China scrambling to limit further person-to-person transmission of the virus, now known as COVID-19.

Wuhan, with a population of 11 million, is under lockdown. Many provinces have postponed the resumption of work at non-essential enterprises following the Chinese New Year holiday, with residents instead staying indoors in barricaded neighborhoods.

Much inter-city and inter-provincial transportation has been halted. And some local governments have even established illegal checkpoints to prevent vehicles carrying industrial products and materials from entering areas under their jurisdiction that contain factories.

The White Swans of 2020

Clearly, the outbreak and the extraordinary official measures to contain it have hit China's economy hard. No one yet knows when the authorities will manage to overcome the epidemic, and what the eventual cost to the economy will be.

But the Chinese people have, once again, shown courage and solidarity in the face of a national emergency. There is no doubt that China will win the battle against COVID-19.

When the severe acute respiratory syndrome (SARS) virus hit the Chinese economy in the spring of 2003, everyone initially was pessimistic about the outbreak's likely economic impact. But as soon as the epidemic was contained, the economy rebounded strongly, and ultimately grew by 10% that year.

China is unlikely to be that lucky this time, given unfavorable domestic and external economic conditions. So, with the deadly coronavirus still on the rampage, the Chinese authorities must prepare for the worst.

Policymakers should respond to the current crisis in three ways. Their first priority must be to rein in the epidemic no matter what the cost. Because markets cannot function properly in emergencies, the state must play the decisive role. Fortunately, China's administrative machinery is functioning effectively.

At the moment, one of the most serious economic obstacles is the interruption to transport caused by fearful local governments. While recognizing local officials' legitimate concerns about preventing the further spread of the virus, the central government must now intervene to facilitate smooth flows of people and materials, thus minimizing supply-chain disruptions.

Second, the government should devise ways to help businesses survive the crisis, focusing in particular on small and medium-size services firms.

While being careful not to create undue moral hazard, the government should cut taxes, reduce charges, and compensate hard-hit enterprises generously. It also should consider establishing pandemic insurance funds so that society as a whole can bear businesses' virus-related losses.

Moreover, commercial banks should strive to ensure that there is no shortage of liquidity, including by rolling over loans to troubled enterprises and allowing them to postpone repayment.

In addition, policymakers may need to resort to market-unfriendly measures such as targeted lending and moral suasion to steer the allocation of financial resources, as well as possibly loosening some financial regulations.

Third, the authorities should pursue more expansionary fiscal and monetary policies, even if such measures *per se* are not aimed at offsetting the negative impacts of supply-side shocks.

The People's Bank of China should continue to lower interest rates as much as possible and inject enough liquidity into the money market. Although inflation has risen as a result of supply-chain disruptions and may yet climb further, tightening macroeconomic policy at this point would be counterproductive.

Likewise, although the government is unlikely to launch large-scale infrastructure investment projects before COVID-19 has been contained, the general budget deficit may nonetheless grow, owing to the epidemic-related increase in spending and decrease in tax revenues.

In its fight to control the virus's spread, the government should not worry too much about whether the budget deficit exceeds 3% of GDP.

The battle against the coronavirus undoubtedly will be very costly, and will reverse some of the Chinese authorities' recent achievements in reining in financial risks.

For now, however, any potential problems related to debt, inflation, or asset bubbles are secondary. Policymakers can worry about them once the situation has calmed down.

Late last year, I sparked a heated debate among Chinese economists by arguing that the country's policymakers should not allow annual GDP growth to slip below 6%, because expectations of a slowdown are self-fulfilling. In the light of the coronavirus outbreak, I concede that the 6% growth target must be reconsidered.

But even if the epidemic lowers growth in 2020 by, say, one percentage point, this probably would not negatively affect people's expectations, because the slowdown would be the result of an external shock rather than some inherent weakness in the economy.

Chinese policymakers' most urgent challenge is no longer how to stimulate aggregate demand, but rather how to ensure that the economy functions as normally as possible without compromising the fight against COVID-19.

Sooner or later, however, the epidemic will be conquered, and the Chinese economy will return to a normal growth path.

When that happens, the question of whether China needs more expansionary fiscal and monetary policies to achieve an adequate level of growth will return to the agenda.

And the rationale for a looser stance will still apply. In fact, to compensate for the losses arising from the COVID-19 outbreak, the Chinese authorities may have to adopt even more expansionary policies than I (and others) had previously suggested.

THE CORONAVIRUS IS JUST STARTING TO HAVE AN IMPACT ON THE GLOBE'S ECONOMY AND POLITICS

The World Health Organization has made it official: Coronavirus is the first "global health emergency" of our new era of major power competition. It will affect global markets, but also geopolitics, as well.

It's already clear that the coronavirus' impact, though too early to fully measure, will be significant on Chinese and global supply chains, markets and economies; on the legitimacy and the trust enjoyed by the Chinese Communist Party with its own people; and on Asian regional politics and U.S.-Chinese relations, where trust already was in such short supply.

So, it's not too early to contemplate the potential, unintended consequences of the virus, thought to have originated in a Wuhan wildlife wet market yet already having resulted in more than 210 deaths and more than 10,000 confirmed cases in 19 regions of China and 20 countries around the world. The cases now include the first person-to-person transmission in the United States, and a rare State Department level four advisory of "do not travel" to anywhere in China.

So even in a heavy news week during which the United Kingdom left the European Union, the United States announced a new Mideast peace plan, and the Senate advanced its impeachment trial of President Trump, none of that beats the potential of coronavirus for global impact.

The first effect, and perhaps the easiest of them all to measure, will be the hit to Chinese and other markets and economies, at a time when the world in any case was wary of a "black swan" event that might nudge it toward recession after the world economy's worst year in a decade in 2019. U.S. markets convulsed Friday, falling by more than 600 points.

The impact is all the greater as it coincides with what was already a slowing Chinese economy. It comes at a time when American and other countries' companies were already shifting supply lines from China to elsewhere due to new tariffs and trade tensions. The virus will serve as another reminder for companies to more rapidly diversify their supply chains.

Following the "phase one" trade deal with the United States, the coronavirus hit also undermines the whiff of bilateral trade optimism that had buoyed markets. It has quickly changed the narrative and increased the odds of a global market downturn in 2020. That's particularly true among emerging markets and investments in commodities from oil to copper, both down double-digits.

Should the crisis stretch out for another month, and experts now consider it more likely than not to reach well into summer, the cost could be a two-percentage point decline in Chinese growth to 4% or lower this year. First quarter growth figures in China could fall to 2% year-on-year – which would be the lowest in decades, and down from 6% in the last quarter of 2019.

The impact on the global economy will be far more significant than during the SARS pandemic of 2003, which is estimated to have provoked a global economic loss of $40 billion and a hit of 0.1% on global GDP. That's because China's share of global GDP has quadrupled since then to 16% from 4% – and fully a third of global growth has been coming from China.

Tourism markets will take an outsized hit, as about 163 million Chinese tourists in 2018 accounted for nearly a third of travel retail sales worldwide. Thailand, for example, has already reduced its 2020 GDP forecast, based on expected revenue losses of as much as $1.6 billion from 2 million fewer Chinese visitors, should travel restrictions continue for a further three months.

More difficult to calculate will be the impact of the virus on Chinese President Xi Jinping's legitimacy and that of his Communist Party.

Wall Street Journal columnist Daniel Henninger referred to a rare public apology by Wuhan's mayor, Zhou Xianwang, as "an epitaph" for the People's Republic of China.

"As a local government official," said the mayor in explaining his slow response, "after I get this kind of information I still have to wait for authorization before I can release it." Wrote Andy Xie in the South China Morning Post: "Wuhan's failure shows up the systemic weaknesses in the top-down structure of the China model, where everyone in the hierarchy is accountable to someone above."

"Though the economy will bounce back when the virus fades," writes The Economist, "the reputation of the Communist party and even of Xi Jinping may be more lastingly affected.

The party claims that, armed with science, it is more efficient at governing than democracies. The heavy-handed failure to contain the virus suggests otherwise."

That brings one to the hardest impacts to calculate of all, and that is the geopolitics of coronavirus.

What's known is that Chinese leaders' confidence in their own rise, and the competitiveness of their alternative authoritarian capitalist economic model grew enormously during and in the aftermath of the global financial crisis of 2008 and 2009.

Could the coronavirus have the reverse impact? The virus may or may not be overblown as a pandemic threat, but Xi's legitimacy in any case will be tested in his handling of the emergency, given how much power has been concentrated in his own hands. Conversely, his authority could grow if he's perceived at handling the crisis well.

Meanwhile, the Atlantic Council's Digital Forensic Research Lab this week spotted what might be a sneak preview of how the global finger-pointing might shift through disinformation should the crisis deepen.

Several narratives have spread first on extreme Russian nationalist sites and to the Chinese internet, blaming the U.S. for the coronavirus outbreak.

They've now been amplified by the Russian mainstream publications Pravda and Izvestiya. It's reminiscent of Operation Infektion, when Russian propaganda during the Cold War tried to pin the spread of the AIDS virus on the United States.

At the same time, the Washington Times quoted a former Israeli military intelligence officer, who has studied Chinese biological warfare, saying that the coronavirus may have originated in an advanced virus research laboratory in Wuhan.

Mercifully, Chinese authorities are taking full responsibility thus far, although without being definitive about the virus' origins, and U.S. officials thus far have praised the efforts.

UNSC MEETING ON COVID-19 INCONCLUSIVE AS US, CHINA ENGAGE IN WAR OF WORDS

A special session of the UN Security Council (UNSC), the decision making body of the United Nations, on the novel coronavirus called overnight Friday seems to have ended inconclusively but not without the US demanding complete transparency and timely sharing of public data, seen as a swipe at China. Beijing on its part hit back saying the spread of covid-19 —which surfaced in China last year – was a "global challenge" and required "cooperation," and "mutual support" to be defeated and not by "scapegoating" anyone. The virus has infected 1.6 million people world over and has claimed 95,731 lives. As of now, the US is the most affected country with over 466,000 infections and a death toll of about 17,000.

The session was called by the current president of the UNSC, the Dominican Republic, in response to requests by nine of the 10 non-permanent members of the Council. And it was the first discussion on the covid-19 pandemic as a threat to world peace and security since the disease surfaced in China in December. Last month, Russia and South Africa had backed China to stall a push by Estonia to initiate a discussion in the UNSC on covid-19. While Russia and South Africa pointed out that there was no direct link between the spread of novel coronavirus and threat to global peace and security, China, the president of the UNSC till 31 March, had rejected the proposal saying that there was no consensus on discussing the matter within the Council. Consensus among members is a key requirement to take up any proposal for discussion and this in turn has led to criticism against the UN for its lack of leadership on matters related to the pandemic.

In her statement US envoy to the UN, Kelly Craft made a pointed reference to the need for transparency, seen as a dig at China, which has been time and again accused of hiding facts about when and how the SARS-Cov2 surfaced and also bring less than transparent about the extent of infections and deaths in the country before it spread around the world. "The United States reiterates today the need for complete transparency and the timely sharing of public health data and information within the international community. The most effective way to contain this pandemic is through accurate, science-based data collection and analysis of the origins, characteristics, and spread of the virus. We cannot stress enough how important these methods are," Craft said.

Craft's call for transparency reiterated the point made by US President Donald Trump and US Secretary of State Mike Pompeo on the need for China to reveal more the origins of the SARS-CoV2 virus that causes covid-19. Both Trump and Pompeo have referred to the pathogen as the "Chinese Virus" or the "Wuhan virus" to underscore its origin in the Chinese city of Wuhan and message that Beijing should have acted faster to warn the world. China's envoy Zhang Jun on his part defended Beijing's record on curbing the spread of infections saying, "Under the leadership of President Xi Jinping and with the utmost sense of responsibility for the Chinese people and people of the world, the Chinese government has adopted the most comprehensive, thorough and strict measures of prevention and control. Important results have been achieved at the current stage."

On its record since the infections spread around the world, Zhang said, "China has provided support of various forms to more than 100 countries, including all those on the agenda of the Security Council, providing medical supplies, sharing experience, sending expert teams and assisting with commercial procurement. China's support will not stop so long as the pandemic is not over."

Zhang also stressed on the need for solidarity among the international community to defeat the challenge. "The COVID-19 pandemic shows once again that people of the world live in a global village and have a shared future," he said. "To overcome this global challenge, solidarity, cooperation, mutual support and assistance is what we need, while beggar-thy-neighbour or scapegoating will lead us nowhere. Any acts of stigmatization and politicization must be rejected." On his part, the UN Secretary-General, Antonio Guterres, urged the UNSC to unite in its response to the covid-19 pandemic, calling it "the fight of a generation — and the 'raison d'etre' of the United Nations itself."

"A signal of unity and resolve from the Council would count for a lot at this anxious time," he told the group adding that the pandemic was the "gravest test" since the UN was founded 75 years ago. After the meeting, the Council issued a short statement, agreed by consensus, which expressed support for Guterres' efforts concerning "the potential impact of Covid-19 pandemic to conflict-affected countries," a Reuters report said.

US GLOBAL RESPONSE TO COVID-19: GOOD INTENTIONS, BAD RESULTS

The United States has conducted, with few positive results, its own disaster diplomacy as COVID-19 spreads, specifically targeting adversaries such as North Korea and Iran. While North Korea did not appear to outright reject the United States' offer of assistance, North Korean leader Kim Jong Un's sister said in a public statement, that such assistance would not improve relations. Iran's Supreme Leader, Ayatollah Ali al Khamenei, more directly refused any US assistance, accusing it of using it to spread the disease. Echoing this sentiment, influential Iraqi Shia cleric Muqtada al Sadr preemptively rejected any vaccines that originated in the United States, despite the fact the virus as a 13 percent fatality rate in Iraq, one of the highest in the world. These examples do not suggest that US assistance has not been well-received elsewhere; however, where it has been, recipients have already had good relations with the United States. Such aid may have been important to reinforcing those relations, but it certainly was not "transformative."

Russia and China's response: Disaster Diplomacy run amok

The United States is not alone in trying to turn crisis into opportunity. Russia and China have also tried to use the pandemic to position themselves as global leaders, often at the expense of the United States. Russia's extremely odd effort to portray a purchase by the United States of ventilators and personal protective equipment (PPE) as "humanitarian assistance" fooled very few. Perhaps even worse, the Italian press criticized Russian aid as "missing the mark" and accused some of the Russian providers of being spies. As a result, while the government did express gratitude for the assistance, it failed to have any transformative effects.

China, on the other hand, has been much more aggressive in its outreach. It has provided funds, doctors, PPE, test kits, and other assistance to numerous countries in Africa, Asia, and Europe. A major reason for this outreach appears to be China's desire to overcome negative publicity associated with its perceived poor handling of the crisis early on, exacerbated by recent reports that the Chinese government waited six days after realizing it had a pandemic on its hands to take steps to curb the spread. By setting itself up as a provider rather than a recipient of aid, it has been able to portray itself as being competent in handling the domestic crisis, since it has excess supplies to send abroad, as well as a valuable partner in combating the global spread. In some other cases, China's interest appears to diffuse broader criticism of its foreign policy. For example, it provided assistance to critics such as Estonia and Lithuania and was able to generate some positive statements suggesting an improvement in relations.

However, its success in bolstering its position as a global leader has, at best, been mixed. While the European Union (EU) did express appreciation for Chinese assistance, EU statements have emphasized the aid's reciprocal nature, often observing the EU provided aid to China as well. In Africa, the reaction appears even more mixed. While a number of African states have expressed gratitude, Nigerian doctors, for example, threatened to cease treating COVID-19 patients if the government invited Chinese doctors to the country. Not only were the Nigerian doctors concerned that the Chinese assistance would "demean their sacrifices" without being effective, they linked the arrival of Chinese doctors in Italy to an increase in cases there. Even worse for the Chinese, there are widespread rumors that the medical equipment it provides is contaminated with the virus.

The pitfalls of Disaster Diplomacy

This last point highlights the pitfalls of trying to use pandemics as political opportunities. Viruses are not earthquakes. In natural disasters it is easier to associate any assistance with relief from a crisis's effects. However, as the Iranian supreme leader's comments and China's experience in Africa indicate, that is not the case in pandemics. Often, aid arrives as the virus is still spreading, all but guaranteeing that it will correlate with higher infection rates and fatalities.

Of course, being aware of this unfortunate perception should not preclude the United States from continuing to provide medical assistance globally. As of March 2020, it has provided $274 million in new assistance to help a number of countries combat the virus. More importantly, the United States provides this assistance through international organizations such as the World Health Organization (WHO) or directly funds responsible agencies in recipient countries. This, however, is a double-edge sword. Following this route allows the United States to avoid the pitfalls of providing assistance directly while preserving its ability to provide critical relief. Of course, doing so also obscures the US role in providing that assistance, diminishing any potential transformative effect.

The way ahead

So while the United States could use a global public relations boost, the wrong moves right now include reducing or discontinuing current levels of assistance, or increasing direct assistance, especially in areas where US intentions are often misunderstood, mistrusted, or easily portrayed as malign. Doing the former would not only exacerbate the crisis, it would enable competitors and critics to portray the United States in a bad light and bring into question intentions behind any future assistance. Perhaps more to the point, given US domestic needs and production capacity, it is not clear if the country can adequately compete in this space. China's ability to produce protective masks, for example, exceeds that of the United States.

There are two areas where the United States can focus its efforts to avoid the pitfalls described above while increasing its chances of achieving transformative effects. First, the United States should look for opportunities where it can free up indigenous resources to combat the virus. For example, as Fred Hof argues, reducing at least some sanctions on Iran would increase the resources Tehran has to combat the virus. Doing so would not only send positive message to the Iranian people of US concern for their well-being, but it would also undermine Tehran's effort to portray the United States as culpable for the virus's spread. Perhaps, more importantly, it will help reduce Iran's role as source of the infection in the region and establish the United States' role as a global partner in combatting the virus, something Iran cannot do. Of course, as Hof notes, there is a high risk that Iranian leadership will misuse some that relief; however, even if they do, that use will only marginally increase Iran and its proxies' effectiveness. Thus, the benefit of relief will likely far outweigh any risks. While any positive message would be undermined by making any relief contingent on political objectives, there could still be an understanding that Iran's cessation of attacks on US forces in Iraq—at least for the duration of the relief—would be a condition for the United States optimizing that relief.

Second, the United States should now consider ways to help critical states with recovery. The World Bank and International Monetary Fund have already urged creditors to provide debt relief to the poorest economies and the Group of Twenty pledged $5 trillion to limit job and income losses. However, even wealthy countries' economies are going to be hard hit, suggesting that there may be insufficient resources to meet the need. This point suggests the importance of getting assistance or relief where it will do the most good, as well as the opportunity to demonstrate the United States' value as a partner.

Bibliography

Andersen, Petter I: *Discovery and development of safe-in-man broad-spectrum antiviral agents*, 2020.

Boulnois, Luce: *Silk Road: Monks, Warriors and Merchants on the Silk Road.* Odyssey Publications, 2005.

Burki, Talha: *Outbreak of coronavirus disease 2019*, 2019.

Chen, W.: *Early containment strategies and core measures for prevention and control of novel coronavirus pneumonia in China*, 2020.

Chen, Yun; Guo, Yao; Pan, Yihang; Zhao, Zhizhuang Joe: *Structure analysis of the receptor binding of 2019-nCoV*, 2020.

Chen, Yusha; Pradhan, Sushmita; Xue, Siliang: *What are we doing in the dermatology outpatient department amidst the raging of 2019-nCoV?*, 2020.

Chun-Han Zhu, *Clinical Handbook of Chinese Prepared Medicines*, Paradigm Publications, Brookline, MA, 1989.

Cyranoski, David: *When will the coronavirus outbreak peak?*, 2020.

Du, B.; Qiu, H. B.: *Pharmacotherapeutics for the New Coronavirus Pneumonia*, 2020.

Dwivedi, G.S., and Mehra, Y.N. : *Ototoxicity of chloroquine phosphate.* Journal of Laryngology and Otology, 1978.

Elisseeff, Vadime: *The Silk Roads: Highways of Culture and Commerce.* UNESCO Publishing. Paris. 1998

Ena, J.; Wenzel, R. P: *A Novel Coronavirus Emerges*, 2020.

Gross, Charles G.: *Brain, Vision, Memory: Tales in the History of Neuroscience.* MIT Press, Delhi, 1999.

Gwaltney JM Jr. *Virology and immunology of the common cold.* Rhinology. 1985

Harding, Harry: *China's Second Revolution.* Washington, DC: Brookings, 1987.

Hollihan, Thomas A. : *Uncivil Wars, Political Campaigns in a Media Age*, Boston: St. Martins, Delhi, 2001.

Huber, G. C.: *Sympathetic Nervous System*, Jour. Comp. Neur., 1897.

Hunt, E. K. *History of Economic Thought, A Critical Perspective*, New York, HarperCollins, 1992.

Ikram, S. M.: *Indian Muslims and Partition of India.* Delhi: Atlantic, 1995.

Imtiaz, A.: *State and Foreign Policy: India's Role in South Asia*, New Delhi, Vikas, 1993.

Jain, U.C. and Jeevan Nair : *Encyclopaedia of Indian Government and Politics*, 2000.

Janowitz, M.: *The Professional Soldier: A Social and Political Portrait*, N.Y., The Free Press, 1960.

Jha, Prem Shankar : *India, America and China : The Battle Between Soft and Hard Power*, Penguin Books India, Delhi, 2010.

Judy A.: *Feminism, Objectivity and Economics,* London and New York, Routledge, 1996.

Kelly, John B.: *Britain and the Persian Gulf 1795-1880*, Oxford, Clarendon Press, 1968.

Keyes K.E. : *Emergency Management for Records and Information Programs,* ARMA International, Kansas, 1997.

Kripalani, Krishna : *All Men are Brothers*, Navjivan Publishing House, 1937.

Kumar, R. and Meenal Kumar : *Prevention of Lifestyle Diseases : Live a Healthy Lifestyle to Fight Diseases*, Deep and Deep, Delhi, 2003.

Laquer, Walter: *Terrorism Attack from Computer Hacking*, Oxford: Oxford University Press, 1999.

Lieberthal, Kenneth: *Governing China*. New York: WW Norton, 1995.

Link, Albert N.: *Evaluating Economic Damages, A Handbook for Attorneys*, Westport, CT, Quorum Books, 1992.

Luo, Hui; Tang, Qiao-Ling: *Can Chinese Medicine Be Used for Prevention of Corona Virus Disease 2019*, 2020.

Magnussen, L., *Evolutionary and Neo-Schumpeterian Approaches to Economics*, Kluwer, Boston, 1994.

Michael Murray: *Heart Disease and High Blood Pressure*, Orient Paperbacks, 2010.

Nandi, N: *Rabies: A Killer Disease*, International Book, Delhi, 2009.

Raman Kapur and Sunita Kapur: *Acupuncture Cure for Common Diseases*, Orient Paperbacks, Delhi, 2001.

Salancik, G. R.: *The External Control of Organizations, A Resource Dependence Perspective*, New York, 1978.

Shikha Saxena: *Phytochemicals and Heart Diseases : Causation and Prevention*, Mittal Publication, Delhi, 2011.

Shirk, Susan L.: *The Political Logic of Economic Reform in China*. Berkeley: University of California Press, 1993.

Singh, Jagbir : *Disaster Management : Future Challenges and Opportunities*, I K Pub, Delhi, 2007.

Smith, V. L.: *Papers in Experimental Economics*, Cambridge, Cambridge University Press, 1991.

Sudeshna Chakravarti: *German Racism : An Old or New Disease*, K.P. Bagchi, Delhi, 1998.

Tietenberg, Tom, *Environmental Economics and Policy,* New York, HarperCollins, 1994

Tinbergen, Jan.: *On the Theory of Economic Policy*, Amsterdam, North-Holland 1952.

Tyagi, B K : *Vector Borne Diseases : Epidemiology and Control*, Scientific, Delhi, 2008.

Upreti, Ganga Dutt: *Proverbs & Folklore of Kumaun and Garhwal*. Lodiana Mission Press, 1894.

Zimmermann, F.M. : *Tourism and Development in Mountain Regions*. Wallingford: CABI Publishing, 2000.

Index

A

Alternative Medicine, 46.

B

Black Swan, 156, 173, 183, 184, 189, 214.

C

China Coronavirus, 83, 128.

Chinese Demand, 1, 160, 163, 175.

Chinese Economy, 157, 159, 176, 180, 182, 185, 186, 208, 210, 212, 213, 214.

Coronavirus Disease, 3, 9, 10, 43, 71, 89, 172, 198.

Coronavirus Intensifies Across Europe, 100.

Coronavirus Outbreak, 3, 5, 16, 17, 38, 51, 55, 57, 61, 72, 73, 81, 82, 95, 97, 98, 140, 142, 156, 173, 184, 186, 199, 206, 208, 210, 219, 220.

Coronavirus Quarantine, 79.

Coronavirus Second Wave, 89.

Coronavirus Spikes, 90.

Coronavirus Surges, 90.

Coronavirus Symptoms, 138, 206.

Coronavirus Treatment, 139.

COVID-19 Fatigue, 117.

COVID-19 Research, 74.

Covid-19 Second Wave Infection, 94.

D

Diagnostic Tests, 150.

Disaster Diplomacy, 218, 219.

Domestic Responses, 15.

E

Economic Effects, 154.

Economic Gloom Worldwide, 185.

Economic Impact, 34, 39, 96, 98, 160, 161, 185, 192, 193, 194, 202, 208, 209, 212.

Epidemiology, 5, 46, 48.

F

First Wave, 92, 93, 97, 98, 99, 100, 101, 103, 106, 107, 109, 112, 118.

Foreign Citizens, 25.

G

Gastrointestinal Tract, 95.

Global Disorder, 187.

Global Economy, 2, 34, 41, 42, 156, 157, 158, 160, 164, 169, 171, 174, 177, 180, 181, 182, 183, 184, 200, 215.

Global Influence, 189.

Global Society, 89.

Global Threat, 125.

H

Hubei Lockdowns, 71.

I

Indian Economy, 97, 99, 183, 194, 200.

Infectious Diseases, 190.

International Responses, 22.

Isolation, 18, 51, 60, 63, 71, 76, 77, 78, 79, 87, 93, 130, 146, 198.

❑❑❑